# Psoriasis Warrior

## The Miracle Program For Clear Skin

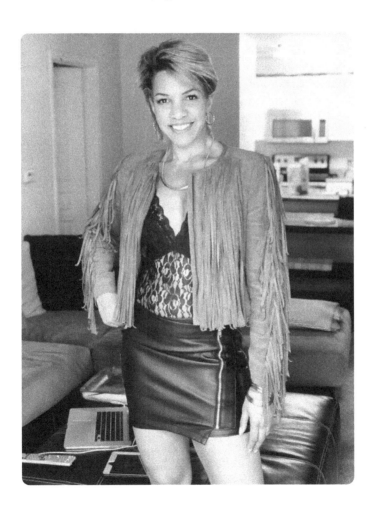

Contact Me : Psoriasistv@gmail.com
www.psoriasiswarrior.com
Facebook – @Psoriasiswarrior
Instagram-@Skinfighters

## Completely Clear and Staying Clear 4 years

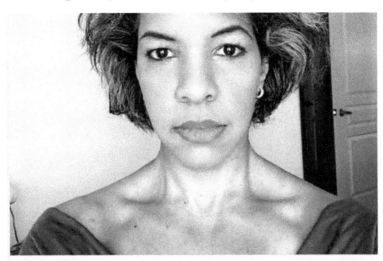

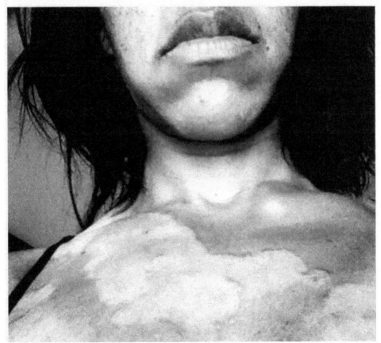

*"The people who are crazy enough to think they can change the world are the ones who often do"- Steve Jobs*

# Foreword

Nothing feels better than beautiful flawless skin. It's no wonder that the skincare industry is worth billions of dollars. I appreciate everyday that my skin is now soft, supple and--best of all--completely clear. For over twenty years, I had the autoimmune condition, Psoriasis which left me looking like a leper. We can hide everything except our skin, so people with skin diseases spend their lives searching for the next medication, cream, shampoo, lotion or pill which will help the flare-ups magically disappear. This was me. Day after day, I could barely focus on anything else. I desperately searched for something to clear my skin. It affected my emotions, my psychology, motivation and depression. Finally, after trying everything possible, every pharmaceutical treatment, every alternative therapy, lotion, cream, pill, spray and herbal treatment, my life changed dramatically, when my skin cleared up completely, using natural healing, only. Today, 4 years later, I am still clear. This was revolutionary, because up til now, I relied on using many drugs –immune suppressants, biological, steroid pills, creams and injections. None of it worked. But, for the first time in more than 20 years, I was using no medications, pharmaceutical drugs or creams and my skin is completely clear and staying clear long-term.

The concept of this unique book is to emphasize the power to heal the body with the help of detoxing, dietary changes, cleansing, exercise, natural supplements, stress management and change of lifestyle. My goal is to help you understand what I think is happening with Psoriasis and what steps you can take to get long-lasting relief, just as I have achieved. This is not going to be a quick-fix or a miracle cure. There is no easy answer for psoriasis or why it happens. But, with the help of making very healthy choices, daily with diet and natural remedies, you will feel and look better, healing your body from the inside out.

I was diagnosed with Psoriasis, when I was only seven years old and when my doctors told me there was no cure, it felt like a death sentence. This may seem exaggerated, but when you learn that you will spend the rest of your life looking disfigured, covered in huge, red, scaly patches, aware of the ugliness of your skin, everyday, and unable to hide or ignore the stares or comments, you feel disillusioned. I wanted to be a model. Ironically, that would never be the path for me. Up until 10 years old, my skin was clear but after this, I was constantly covered all through teenage and adult life with large, unsightly patches of Psoriasis.

## Psoriasis On My Scalp In Childhood

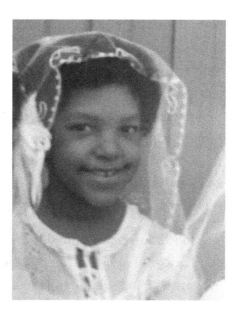

In many ways, people with skin diseases are stuck leading a life of solitude because of the challenge of dealing with the symptoms--itchy, red, scaly skin--but, also the emotional toll it takes to live everyday with breakouts. No one understands this challenge more than me. Psoriasis affected every aspect of living. I had few friendships, fewer relationships and I felt like an outcast every day for over twenty years. No swimming, play-dates, sleepovers or prom. I was forbidden to interact with many of my peers as they feared that they would contract this horrible skin disease. Every day of my childhood was an absolute nightmare. It took pure courage to even go to school and endure, horrid treatment. I felt alienated, alone and depressed.

Day after day. I was consumed with one thought – how to get rid of it. I read, research, sought doctors, naturopaths, dermatologists and natural healers – anyone who could point me in the right direction. I was obsessed with the idea that there had to be a potential treatment which would clear my skin forever. After exhausting all avenues, I abandoned the search for a pill or medication and began to investigate natural healing. I put into practice every possible home remedy I found. Then one day, after years of searching, hope came to me when I discovered the healing power of detoxing, dietary changes and natural healing.

Though the concept was new to me, natural healing and the power of food is not new. As far back as 1210 AD, Hippocrates said, "Let food be thy medicine and medicine be thy food." As much as skin conditions like psoriasis are frustrating to people who battle them daily, they cannot be ignored. Skin diseases tend to be related to imbalances with systems in the body. Psoriasis is still part of the autoimmune family of medical diseases and doctors agree that involves the immune system and inflammation together with the digestive system and liver. It requires medical care by a qualified physician. That said, the decision to pursue natural approaches like cleansing, detox, diet and stress management is not wrong. Medications and pharmaceutical drugs have dangerous side effects, which can have long-term consequences. I took them dutifully for almost my entire life and it result in very little change for my skin. In addition, the cost of drugs are increasing and many people, including me, are simply are not financially able to finance the thousands of dollars that drug plans cost. I have many stories, including my own, of people who have been driven to bankruptcy, lost their houses, their spouses and dramatically reduced the quality of their lives because of the thousands of dollars –sometimes up to $50,000 a year in expenses on pharmaceutical drugs. For a skin condition as unpredictable as Psoriasis, this burden seems never-ending. Picture never being able to follow your dreams because the look of your skin hinders you and you are deathly afraid that it will get worst. I had a childhood dream or being a model or a journalist. As I got older, the realization that this would never happen, propelled me into applied sciences with chemical engineering. However, this too would be short lived as the chemicals I was coming into contact with made my skin worst. Then, I had an interest in fitness, but Psoriatic arthritis began to affect my joints, muscles and movements so I was in pain every day. I gave up track and field as a child, gymnastics and all sports. Psoriasis destroyed so much of my ability to live a normal life.

This was my situation. I was depressed, disillusioned, gaining massive amounts of weight and I felt like a failure. Drug after drug failed, leaving me covered head to toe in outbreaks, year after year.

## Psoriasis Flare Ups While Using Medications

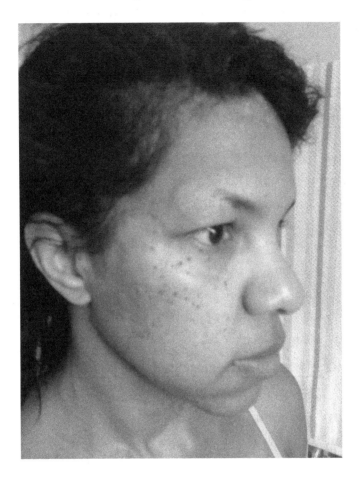

Sometimes I would go months with hope, watching it slowly fade, only to wake up, one morning with a complete change where patches spread out of control. I was driven into complete isolation sometimes, having to go to the hospital because it became unmanageable.

The lowest point for people with Psoriasis is when you become suicidal and you feel like you cannot live another day, in so much pain. It's a constant daily battle that many doctors and dermatologists do not understand. So, with no hope people with Psoriasis and Psoriatic Arthritis never feel motivated to see their physicians and tend to stop going. I felt this way too.

One day, I just got so fed up, I decided to pursue the alternative healing route. It was not easy. I had to learn everything I could about nutrition, health anatomy, physiology and naturopathy. But, over twenty years, all of this information, as well as a change in diet, supplements and lifestyle led to my being 100% clear of psoriasis with no pain from psoriatic arthritis, and I did it in less than eight weeks. When something like natural healing changes your life and the lives of thousands of others, it cannot be ignored. This is my attempt to tell my story in hopes that it will help the millions of people with skin conditions, who want to see change. My wish is that this book gives you hope to know that you are not alone and that you can see and feel substantial change in your skin and your health just by making a few changes and supporting the healing process.

Few people can understand living with a condition involving misinformation and dozens of medications and creams which claim to work. Some show promise at first, but after a couple of months, they stop working and cause flare-ups. Worst yet, problem skin has now become the industry plagued by scam products and marketing of everything from herbal pills to a witch's brew to clear the skin. In desperation we turn to children's lotions and shampoos, herbal creams, teas, and we fall for every possible remedy fed to us by affiliates of products who have never experienced what its like to have scales and spots growing at an alarming rate. I've had so many people message me over and over with all sorts of remedies, which not only fail but can be dangerous for health. People with psoriasis must deal with this every day of their lives for years and sometimes a lifetime. I was one of these people. I could not walk down the street or sit in a restaurant without people staring, pointing and approaching me to sell something. It was frustrating and pushed me into hiding and depression. Something had to change and it drove me to leave no stone unturned until I found a solution. I was prepared to study, research and learn about everything I could do to find a solution. That's what I did for years.

I travelled the world in search of something that could help me. Consulted with with gurus, doctors, researchers and naturopaths. I know my friends and family probably thought I went mad, but skin conditions can drive you to do very adventurous and downright crazy things. After spending all this time and money researching with health practitioners in North America, Central America, Asia and the Caribbean, I came to see that all healers, including doctors, know that the ability to heal lies inside. So, I questioned gurus, gathered the research, facts and knowledge I gained, after years of meeting some of the greatest authorities in functional and alternative medicine and combined it with my own two and one-half years of study of natural healing at Canadian School of Natural Nutrition, CSNN in Toronto, Canada and I set out to heal myself. It would be one of the most difficult undertakings. Each day, I would study and apply what I learned. There were so many times, Psoriasis spiraled out of control but eventually, I got it right. I was so excited when I first cleared my skin completely, I took to You Tube and created my first set of videos. I was on a mission to help as many people as I could. Four years later . I have helped thousands of people in their journey, to heal their skin. I am honored to say that 95% of them cleared their skin and remain clear today. I have hundreds of stories on Facebook and Instagram, and testimonials from people whose lives have changed dramatically. I am very far from being done.

## 2016 - I First Healed Completely

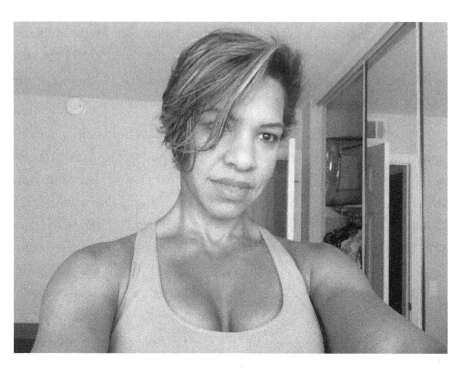

Today I am proud to show that I am 100% clear of psoriasis and staying clear. Best if all, I have hundreds of pictures and videos to show the evidence of my transformation. My skin is clear, glowing and blemish free from changes in diet, natural supplements, changes in lifestyle and hydration. I have documented it all. The irony is that now, I get compliments daily on social media on how beautiful my skin look and I am overjoyed.

So, I ventured to write this book and document this journey. My book is going to get straight to the point. I will share my experience of dealing with psoriasis and how I was finally able to achieve clear skin, using only detox, change of diet and natural remedies. If you are like me, you are at the point where you need a roadmap. That's what this book will provide. Modern medical treatment, medications, pills, injections and steroids have their purpose, and you should discuss all options with your doctor before deciding which to pursue. The goal of this book is to provide you with ways to support your body's own ability to heal using natural remedies which, in my case led to clear skin. I would like to make it clear that I am not a medical professional and this is not considered medical advice. If you are using medications and trying to treat Psoriasis, I strongly suggest you discuss anything you are doing or thinking about trying with your doctor and request direction every step of the way.

This book highlights my own experience helping thousands of people, including myself, to clear their skin. But, it in no way, is it considered a cure as there is no known cure for Psoriasis. Each person is individual and therefore what works for one person or even hundreds may not work everyone. That said, natural healing is one of the best ways to help to manage chronic skin conditions like Psoriasis and it can give complete long-term relief as is shown by thousands of people who have healed. Natural healing addresses the source of the problem, not just suppressing the symptoms. As soon as I took my focus off the appearance of my skin, and moved it to what was happening inside my body and made changes to my diet, digestion, stress management, sleep and overall well-being, I saw a massive transformation occur in my skin and overall health. So while it is impossible to approach healing as a quick-fix, this book will help you to support the healing process with natural steps which will help to improve the look of your skin and potentially clear your skin for good. It is my genuine hope that each and every person who reads this book is inspired and motivated to do everything possible to support the healing of your body. I used this journey as a way to understand my own body and how it responded to healthy habits. I believe that Psoriasis is a warning that our systems are not functioning properly. Later, I discuss the role of immune system, inflammation, liver and detox systems together with stress and neurological function. The body's systems are all interconnected so, when we approach healing from the inside out, it is important to look at all of the systems involved as well as our own lifestyle. By healing the body holistically, we heal the skin and improve overall health. Healing Psoriasis naturally will not only improve the look of your skin, it will change your life. Get ready to analyze and look at everything you are eating, taking and doing daily. I found that the answer lies in what is going into the body and how our bodies are reacting to this. Psoriasis is more prevalent with people who have the autoimmune genes and we will always have Psoriasis. But, natural healing allowed me to have clear skin and no pain. I can live normal without hiding my skin. As a Psoriasis Warrior all of my life, it is my hope that this book helps you with your own healing journey and I encourage you to share this information with your medical doctors and others who are supporting you in your healing.

# Table of Contents

Foreword............................................................................v

Chapter 1: Introduction........................................... 1

Chapter 2: What Is Psoriasis?............................... 10

Chapter 3: The Leaky Gut Syndrome................... 23

Chapter 4: Psoriasis and the Liver....................... 37

Chapter 5: Psoriasis and Stress ............................ 44

Chapter 6: Common Treatments For Psoriasis ... 49

Chapter 7: Transitioning To Natural Healing...... 51

Chapter 8: Natural Healing .................................. 66

Chapter 9: Other Remedies for Natural Psoriasis Healing .............. 82

Chapter 10: Introducing Dietary Changes .......... 87

Chapter 11: The Role of Lifestyle Change ........... 99

Chapter 12: The Psoriasis Detox Diet ................. 104

# CHAPTER 1

## Introduction

I have been a Psoriasis Warrior for over twenty years and during this time, I embarked on a journey to uncover a natural solution which could clear my skin 100% and allow me to lead a normal life. I discovered that it is possible to heal from the inside out and clear the skin completely. I learned this after years of trial and error on my own body; dedicated study in holistic nutrition and naturopathy along with four years helping thousands of people heal psoriasis. I have painstakingly documented this journey and gathered countless testimonials from people worldwide who had psoriasis, and today they are enjoying the freedom that comes with looking in the mirror and instead of seeing plaques, they see their own clear, beautiful skin. But before I could begin this healing journey, I had to get to the point of no return. In 2013, I got to that point. After years of battling psoriasis, I awoke to one of the worst flare-ups ever. My skin was red and painful and thick plaques covered my face. I'd had enough. I had done everything I was advised. I was tired and fed up from taking all the medications prescribed to me, only to have psoriasis cover 80% of my body.

The current medical system failed me. Countless doctors, dermatologists and pharmaceutical drugs didn't seem to help, and I believe they worsened my health and my skin. I couldn't understand how the medical community could be incapable of giving relief to 125 million psoriasis warriors around the world. When I began speaking to people daily about psoriasis, I heard similar stories. These people used drugs, steroids and creams with no change in the skin.

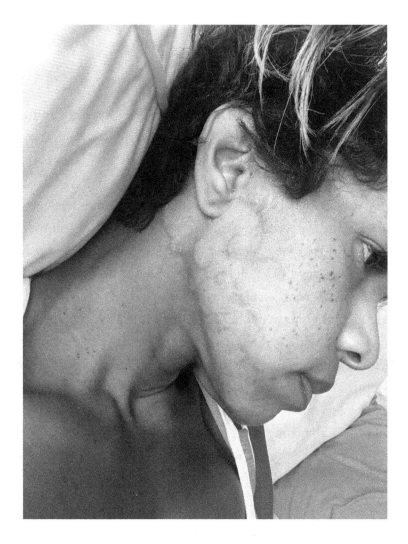

Go on Facebook where groups of people complain daily of side effects like nausea, hair loss, mouth sores, insomnia, chest pain and this does not include the painful, burning and itchy skin that most psoriasis sufferers are forced to live with. I couldn't understand why so many drug companies, skincare companies and natural healers could offer no long-term relief. I was left feeling depressed and defeated every day of my life. I felt hopeless and I locked myself away from the world every chance I got. All along, I knew, in my gut that there was a connection between the state of my skin and my diet. I began to monitor what I was eating 10 years ago. Theories about leaky gut were beginning to emerge and I witnessed that my skin looked less red and less scaly when I ate more vegetables and fruit, and it was more red and inflamed when I ate pizza, burgers and fries. These results propelled me to look deeply into diet and how it was affecting my skin.

I began to read research about how food could affect the digestive system and the bulk of the immune system lay in the gut. I made the connection that if Psoriasis is related to the immune system and a large part of the immune system was in the digestive system, this could be where it begins. I figured if I could stop the effects at the source, then perhaps it could prevent the chain of reactions which ended with Psoriasis outbreaks spreading all over my body. I completed hundreds of food logs and took pictures of my skin every few weeks to try to find a connection between what I was eating and the state of my skin. I wanted to understand why eating certain things caused psoriasis to go out of control. I witnessed these constant flare ups particularly after I ate processed junk food and drank alcohol for weeks. These outbreaks were red, painful and they would spread out of control to cover major parts of my body.

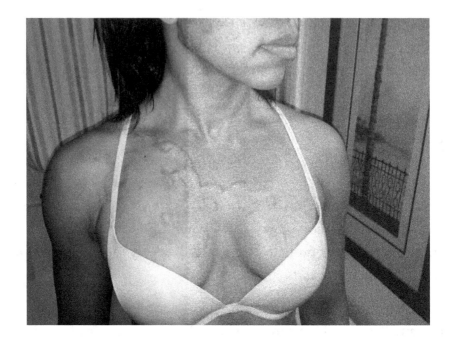

When I eliminated some foods, the opposite would occur. So I discussed with my doctor my diet and the potential connection to clearing my skin. After all, that's what I wanted. I didn't really care about the theories and the reasons no one had found the answer to autoimmune illness. I just wanted to live a normal life. But every time I asked my doctor about the connection between food, diet, and psoriasis, I was shut down and told that there was no evidence of a connection and I should just take drugs. However, living with horrendous side effects was not worth it to me and psoriasis drugs cost the equivalent of a year's salary. All of this pushed me towards a natural solution. I was stubborn and I refused to listen to the several doctors I had over the years. Yes, I switched so many times, in desperation, I lost count. And for the next ten years I began a systematic trial and error of removal and re-introduction of foods until I got it right and I was seeing improvements. I made changes to my stress levels and sleep. I incorporated daily exercise along with meditation. I tried every supplement which even remotely could provide relief and documented changes in my skin. Then, finally, one day in 2016, armed with all of this information, I knew I was close to a breakthrough. I created my Psoriasis Detox Diet program, followed it for seven weeks and there was, what I considered to be a miraculous change. My skin was completely clear. No scars or marks. No more Psoriasis outbreaks on my skin. All signs of psoriasis vanished. I was finally completely clear of psoriasis–no medications, steroid creams or herbal medicines. I felt free. I began to join groups and connect with others who had experienced the same thing. Thousands of people were on the natural path and achieving amazing long lasting results. I spoke to at least 10 people a day, day after day, observing and discussing their progress. I created social media to discuss and document their stories all in the aim of promoting and spreading awareness of natural healing. For the first time in over 20 years, I along with thousands of Psoriasis Warriors, people who felt hopeless and desperate, saw real results following natural healing. It was evident that dietary changes which is at the heart of my program, made a tremendous difference in the healing of my skin.

My concern was, why had my doctors refused to believe that diet had any effect on Psoriasis. For years, I was told, over and over, that what I was eating had absolutely no effect on Psoriasis and changing my diet would not work. Yet, here I was, completely clear and thousands of people were experimenting with changes in diet and getting life-changing results with their skin clearing up.

Then, later, I understood that medical professionals were not wrong in their belief that diet does not cure psoriasis. It's true there is no cure for psoriasis and it's true there is no evidence to suggest that there is any connection between someone's diet and psoriasis outbreaks. Yet, here I am completely clear after I made dietary changes. And I remain clear even today. So why the disconnect? I wondered about this as I continued to help many people do the same thing–change their diet, follow natural healing and clear the skin completely. Why did this evidence of clear skin contradict the opinion of the medical community? Then one day, it hit me. What I was essentially going through--dietary changes and natural healing--was cleansing and detoxing my body. I was also cutting back on many of the processed and packaged foods which we know are laden with chemicals, preservatives and pesticides.

Clean food, proper hydration, essential nutrients and supplementation were crucial parts of a detox and cleansing program. So where diet may not cure psoriasis, cleansing the body and eating plant-based natural foods helps to support the healing process. This series of daily actions helped me to detoxify my body and the actions support the healing of the body and the skin. I had essentially created a detox program. It's no surprise because detoxification has been around for centuries and many of the forefathers of natural medicine believed in the power of cleansing to renew the body and significantly improve health. In the last ten years, toxins and pollution have increased by one hundred times what it was fifty years ago and our bodies are not equipped to deal with so much toxicity. Only recently has research found that psoriasis is related to toxicity and the liver. Doctors are always reminding psoriasis sufferers to have the liver checked. Why ? The main reason is that medications have side effects, which are known to affect the liver. But more importantly, the liver is one of the main organs at the center of psoriasis. I also learned that the liver and skin have an intimate relationship. Since Psoriasis manifests on the skin, it's ironic that the role of the skin is a backup detox organ, and when the liver is overloaded, often the skin will be affected. So, I wasn't surprised when, after years of living with psoriasis outbreaks covering my body, my skin would clear up completely following my Psoriasis Detox Diet program.

Does this mean I cured psoriasis? No, there is no known cure. However, what I proved with my experience and with thousands of people who have discovered the same, is that cleansing, dietary changes and natural remedies work to clear the skin long term. I have been clear for four years with no patches of psoriasis on my skin. Just doing a few daily, natural practices and eating clean nutritious food, drinking lots of water and managing stress can improve the appearance of the skin and make psoriasis disappear. I have come to the realization that psoriasis is a daily care project. Just as we take time to investigate the best way to invest our money for our future, similar investment and investigation into health is required to manage psoriasis.

I found that everything I consumed could affect psoriasis because our digestive system is intimately related to the immune system, the liver and the skin. It makes sense that when we smoke and consume known toxic food, water, medications, pollution, alcohol, it increases inflammation, triggers the immune system, and affects our system. The liver is the main organ which becomes overloaded with toxins and is responsible for removing and making sure that these toxic, harmful chemicals do not circulate in the body. So my theory was that if the liver is responsible for removing toxins, and we are consuming foods and drink with toxins in them which could be overloading the liver and affecting the skin, then cutting back on processed foods and changing the diet, should help the liver and the skin.

This makes sense because most people with psoriasis know that when psoriasis flares up, there is a trigger. The two major triggers of psoriasis--alcohol and smoking--have also been found to be two of the greatest destroyers of the liver and health. It is no surprise that just these two

So with all of these connections, I knew that cleansing and detoxing the body was the solution to alleviating stress on the liver, which could give the skin the opportunity to heal. I was right. By following my Psoriasis Detox Diet program for under eight weeks, I was able to achieve clear skin and I remain clear today.

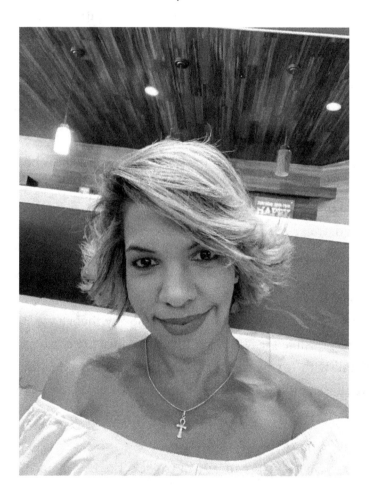

I successfully fought the psoriasis war and won. I'm a true Psoriasis Warrior and I am so excited to share everything I did with others, in hopes that millions of Psoriasis Warriors worldwide can also get relief. This book does not replace your doctor. In fact, just as I have done, I would like you to insist that your doctor read this book along with you so that you are keeping him or her in the loop as to everything you are doing. I am sharing with you my personal journey and the information in this book should never be taken as a diagnosis, treatment or cure. We will always have psoriasis, but we can have clear skin too and we can heal from the inside out. My hope is that by following my program, you too will experience similar effects of completely clear skin and you can use this as a tool for managing Psoriasis for life. My Clear Skin program has also been shown to not only improve the appearance of my skin but it completely transformed my health and well-being. I am happier, healthier and more confident and it has dramatically improved my quality of life and I know it will do the same for you.

# CHAPTER 2

# What Is Psoriasis?

Psoriasis is an autoimmune disease. It is not a skin disease; rather, it is a disease affecting the skin, and it occurs when skin cells are multiplying at a much faster rate than normal. Research shows that the problem begins in the immune system's T cells, which cause abnormal inflammation that leads to a proliferation of skin cells. The exact cause of psoriasis is not yet known, but scientists believe that it is linked to genetics, the immune system, and the environment.

Over the years, I witnessed my psoriasis fade, and then one day, out of the blue, it would return and spread out of control. This is the flare-up stage, and often it is believed to be preceded by a trigger which launches the whole process, and results in outbreaks. This can occur in childhood as was my case, or it can happen in an outbreak later in life in the mid-twenties or thirties, and for some it can even begin in the fifties or sixties.

The trigger can be many things including medications, alcohol, smoking, and chemicals along with excessive stress. This makes psoriasis unpredictable. An outbreak can occur anywhere and it can be a small patch or it can spread out of control to cover 90% of the body. Psoriatic disease can be just as interesting because it can manifest only as pain with or without the skin outbreaks.

Most psoriasis warriors like me live in fear every day, because when the skin begins to clear, it seems at any moment it can stop healing and spread out of control for no apparent reason. I experienced this so many times over 20 years. I would make changes, see my skin improving, and then one day, I would wake up and my body would be eighty percent covered red, scaly, blistering patches.

Psoriasis has also been linked to leaky gut, a condition where the digestive system becomes permeable allowing food particles, bacteria, chemicals and pollution to get into the blood and increase inflammation. Since it is the job of the immune system to hunt down foreign invaders, it mistakes these particles to be invaders and begins to attack them. Many believe that this is the connection between, leaky gut, the immune system, inflammation and the liver. Psoriasis can affect any race, age and sex, although it is more common in the adult population simply because that is when it is diagnosed. There is reduced quality of life because the skin outbreaks affect social life and self-esteem.

The current treatment of psoriasis is always aimed at the skin and shutting down the immune system. Both create additional problems long-term. Psoriasis can be accompanied by pain and this is known as psoriatic arthritis. I had both psoriasis and PSA, so along with outbreaks all over my body, I experienced intense pain daily in my joints like my knees and back. Why psoriasis manifests in both forms is still unknown and it is difficult to get a clear diagnosis for psoriatic arthritis as it is often misdiagnosed as rheumatoid arthritis, for which medications are always prescribed. I believe that these medications make it even more difficult to pursue natural healing, so often, people with psoriasis are stuck taking these drugs for life. It should be noted that psoriatic arthritis can present with pain and no skin outbreaks, which makes it even harder to determine that it is indeed psoriasis.

All of these unknowns make psoriasis a mystery. Still today, I feel that the medical community is no closer to offering long-term hope to the millions of people who are suffering. Its one thing to live with a skin disease; its much harder to deal with the feeling that you can never be one hundred percent free of psoriasis and live a normal life.

## Types of Psoriasis

There are several types of psoriasis all of which have a visible appearance. The following table shows the known types of psoriasis.

| NAME | DESCRIPTION |
|------|-------------|
| Plaque psoriasis | Plaque psoriasis is characterized by patches of red, scaly skin on different areas of the body. Most people with psoriasis at some point suffer with plaque psoriasis. I had it covering 85% of my body for many years. |
| Guttate | Guttate psoriasis appears as small red spots on the skin. Spots can be in one localized area or they can spread to cover the entire body. Guttate often appears after strep throat, stress, surgery or with the use of some medications. |

| NAME | DESCRIPTION |
|---|---|
| Inverse | Inverse psoriasis is characterized as patches in skin folds. It's usually found under breasts, in the groin or in armpits. This form was very uncomfortable for me because there is burning, and it is difficult to keep dry. |
| Palmoplantar | Pustular psoriasis looks like white bumps filled with pus near or inside red skin blotches. There are three types: palmoplantar pustulosis, which generally forms on hands or feet; acropustulosis which tends to be found on fingertips and von zumbusch which are red, painful outbreaks over a wide area of the body. |
| Scalp | Scalp psoriasis shows up as flakes or large red patches over the scalp that can spread down the neck and forehead. |
| Erythrodermic | Erythrodermic psoriasis involves the entire skin and leads to reddening with scaly sheets of skin layers. |

| NAME | DESCRIPTION |
|------|-------------|
| Psoriatic arthritis | Psoriatic arthritis can occur with many other forms or alone. It affects joints with pain in fingers, knees, shoulders and sometimes the back and ankles. |

Approximately 7 million people in North America and over 125 million worldwide have some form of psoriasis and this is growing. Diagnosing this disease can be difficult as many other skin conditions look very similar. What sets psoriasis apart is that there is no cure and--in my experience--many factors can very quickly make it worse. Unless attention to healing from the inside out begins at the start, most people with psoriasis will battle it for life; however, the good news is that more and more research is emerging about natural ways to manage the condition.

## The Immune System's Role in Psoriasis

The role of the immune system is very important to protecting the body from foreign invaders, but it is the immune system's over-reacting, which eventually leads to psoriasis outbreaks. The immune system is a collection of billions of cells that travel through the bloodstream. They are responsible for defending against foreign bodies such as bacteria, viruses and cancerous cells.

There are two types of immune cells:

- B cells produce antibodies which are released into the fluid surrounding the body's cells to destroy the invading viruses and bacteria.

- T cells lock on to the infected cell, multiply and destroy it. These are white blood cells called lymphocytes and the other cells are phagocytes.

Antigens are substances which are recognized by antibodies. A specific antibody is produced to match an antigen. Antigens are usually a protein or polysaccharide, which are the building blocks of sugar.

The US National Library of Medicine states that an antigen can also be a chemical, bacteria or virus. This makes sense since I have seen that all my forms of psoriasis seemed to be triggered by strep, which is a bacterial infection, toxic chemicals, medications and smoking. In general antibodies will match a specific antigen, but there are times where they can bond to several different antigens. So, the way I understand this, is that people with psoriasis like me have created all of these antibodies that will start reacting to lots of different things, which is why the immune system is always in overdrive. It's no wonder that the first thing doctors try to do is suppress the immune system and shut it off, but for me--when we suppress the immune system to calm psoriasis down--it's the same as shutting off our house alarm which was tripped, even though the intruder is still in the house. Suppression only shuts off the alarm; it does not prevent the burglar or intruder from affecting us. In the same way, when we shut down the immune system, we get short-term relief, but we never figure out why the immune system is being triggered.

For over a decade of taking a number of medications, it made no sense to me to attack this problem by simply shutting down my immune system. As I understood it, the immune system serves the very important function of protecting the body in the case of a major foreign invader like a virus, bacteria or parasite. It must mount a response against foreign invaders like viruses and bacteria, but if it's not able to do this job, we are vulnerable to much worse than psoriasis. Unfortunately, psoriasis is an auto-immune condition meaning the immune system is also attacking itself as well as outside environmental triggers, which then contribute to skin outbreaks.

An overactive immune system leads to inflammation as immune cells and complexes bind the cells of the body. Researchers are yet to figure out why this happens, so there is no cure for psoriasis. The reason I chose to follow natural healing was I wanted to get to the source of the problem, instead of shutting down part of the problem for a short-term response. No one knows why we have psoriasis, but over years of trial and error, I could see that controlling and preventing toxic food, drink chemicals and medications produced a transformative change in my health, which I believe contributed to the clearing of my psoriasis. This is why I decided to make dietary changes. It is true there is no scientific research linking psoriasis to diet; however, cleaning up the diet does two major things:

1. Removes inflammatory substances and toxic substances, which overload the body's detox systems; the substances also increase inflammation and send the immune system into overdrive.

2. Provides nutrients in their purest forms to help with the healing of tissues. My experiment worked. After twenty years, my skin is clear; I eat normally and I live a normal life.

## Psoriasis and Inflammation

Psoriasis is also related to inflammation, which is a response to damage in the body. With psoriasis the inflammation is long-term and chronic. Inflammation can affect many parts of the body including joints, the heart and kidneys which is why psoriasis can be related to psoriatic arthritis, which manifests as pain in the joints, cardiovascular disease, diabetes and high blood pressure.

Inflammation is made worse when immune T-cells become involved. The immune system is triggered, and this begins the cascade of processes which lead to outbreaks on the skin. There is also a connection between psoriasis, psoriatic arthritis and inflammatory bowel disease (IBD) which are all linked to inflammation. Research shows that 1 in 10 people with psoriasis are at risk to also have IBD which means that colon health is crucial to managing psoriasis. IBDs like ulcerative colitis and Crohn's disease can cause many symptoms, including abdominal pain, diarrhea, and cramps. Both psoriasis and IBD are related to inflammation and an overactive immune system. Ulcerative colitis mainly affects the lining of the colon and the rectum. Inflammation causes swelling and sores called ulcers to develop in those areas of the digestive tract. Crohn's disease also involves inflammation and ulcers. They can occur anywhere in the digestive tract, but they most commonly affect the small and large intestines. In Crohn's disease, the inflammation can occur much deeper in the intestine lining than is the case with ulcerative colitis symptoms. It is interesting that psoriasis is related to cardiovascular disease, which is also related to inflammation. Psoriatic arthritis presents with increased inflammation leading to pain, so inflammation seems to be a central theme with psoriasis.

## The Skin

Psoriasis presents with spots or patches of outbreaks on the skin. These skin outbreaks develop because as inflammation increases and the immune system is triggered, a series of reactions is set off with white blood cells and eventually the skin is affected. In my experience, anything I put on the skin did not clear psoriasis long term and sometimes the medications like steroid creams had serious side effects and made it spread out of control for years. I also believe that synthetic creams and lotions can be toxic to the skin. Even though the skin is known as the protective barrier and is made up of dead cells, just beneath the outer layer is a layer of living cells, blood supply and nerves.

To understand why psoriasis plaques are formed, it's important to understand what happens to the skin. The skin is an organ which is constantly evolving. There are two layers; the outer layer is the epidermis and the inner layer is the dermis. Cells are formed and mature in the dermis and move to the outer layer, the epidermis where they die and form the outer layer. Psoriasis plaques are formed when the inner dermis are producing cells at a very fast rate so they don't have time to die and form the dead layer.

In psoriasis, the skin turnover is increased to as much as ten times the normal rate. The excess turnover of dead cells lying on the skin's surface are cells which have not yet turned into the dead layer, so they form the red plaque formation with white scales. Because the patches do not have the dead layer, the danger for people with psoriasis is that the inner tissues are now exposed to toxins from the environment and anything we put on the skin. I believe that toxic creams, lotions and medications can get into our blood supply joining all the other toxins coming from the intestines and overloading the body. What you put on your cells can interact with the body's systems by getting absorbed into the blood and traveling around to different organs. This includes steroids and creams with synthetic chemicals.

One look at anatomy and we can see that the skin is only a part of the issue with psoriasis. It is the final part of the solution. It is not the source of the problem; therefore, spending thousands of dollars on creams and lotions for the skin, only results in short-term help or no effect at all. I found it was important to be very careful about what goes on the skin as it is absorbed into the blood. People with psoriasis don't just have spots on their body; these are like open wounds. When the plaques are red and inflamed, this means all of our body's systems are under stress and fighting inflammation and dealing with the effects of an immune system on overdrive.

A major function of the skin is sweating and removal of toxins. The skin is the backup detoxing organ, so when our internal detoxing organs are overloaded, the body turns to the skin to remove toxins. Why detoxing organs become overloaded is still a mystery. People with psoriasis cannot handle the same toxic load as others and organs become overloaded much faster. The fact that the skin is involved in psoriasis suggests that toxins are being removed using the skin and maybe interacting with the cells of the skin.

Research shows that there are higher levels of certain bacteria and inflammation, which seems to affect the immune system. This has been my experience as well. When my body was more toxic, psoriasis plaques spread much faster and they were red and inflamed. I noticed that many times after I had done a detox, my skin improved dramatically, which is how I realized that cleansing the body gently was extremely important. I emphasize gently because if you decide to use over-the-counter detox kits, the detoxing and cleansing process can get too intense and can cause psoriasis plaques to flare out of control because the detox process with these kits can be too aggressive. The cleansing of the body must include cleansing the colon, detox organs and increasing circulation altogether so the body does not try to throw all toxins onto the skin. One theory is that psoriasis tends to appear where there are greater concentrations of sweat glands; as the body tries to get toxins out, these areas develop psoriasis plaques more readily. However, in my experience, I have had full body psoriasis flare-ups where my entire body was covered in psoriasis.

Since the source of psoriasis is internal, in my experience, creams which are the most popular prescribed treatment don't seem to solve the problem. My concern was always long-term clearance of the skin. I was fed up and frustrated by short-term remedies, which helped to clear the skin for a few weeks only to have it spread again and again.

## A Couple Of Weeks Using Natural Healing

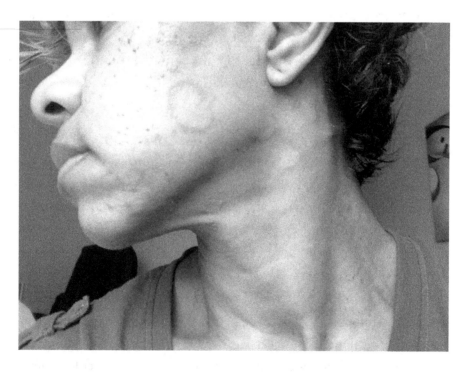

I wanted more than just a few weeks of my skin being clear, and I was anxious about the thought of using toxic substances on my skin that could later affect my health. Not everyone, though, is affected by side effects of creams or medications. Some people have been able to use medications for 20 or 30 years, and it becomes a part of their daily routine. This is still one of the most widespread solutions offered by doctors. However, I personally could not handle the day-to-day struggle of dealing with the numerous effects like nausea, weight-gain, headaches, muscle aches, muscle cramps, dizziness, frequent colds and foggy brain. I was also very concerned with the long-term impact of using medications on my body and health. To me, if psoriasis begins with a trigger like stress, overloaded liver or strep infection, these are all occurring internally. So, putting creams on the skin or taking medications which shut down natural reactions like the immune or inflammatory system made no sense to me. As far as I understood, I need my immune system to function and protect my body against real invaders, so shutting it down was very scary to me. In addition, inflammation is a natural process in the body, so using medications to suppress this too, did not offer hope to clear my skin and live a normal, healthy life. Natural healing does none of these destructive things to the body, so it seemed to be the right path for me.

# Before and After Using Natural Remedies

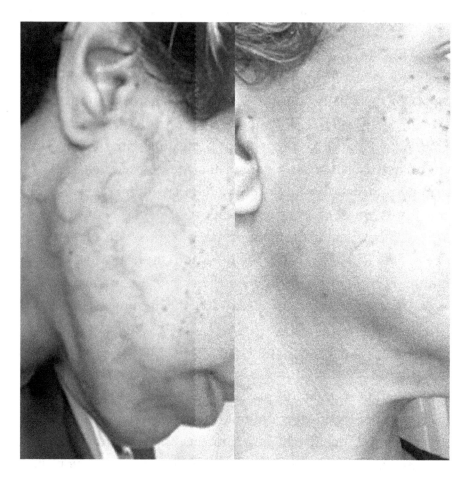

# CHAPTER 3

# The Leaky Gut Syndrome

Since most people with psoriasis experience effects with changes in diet there may be a connection between the digestive system and psoriasis. New research seems to suggest that intestinal permeability and leaky gut could be at the source of the outbreaks. I first learned about this from Dr. Pagano almost twenty years ago in his book *Healing Psoriasis*. Being a pioneer of natural healing of psoriasis he suggested that psoriasis was merely toxins getting into the blood and the body's reaction to this is to trigger the immune system to deal with this foreign matter. Today many things contain toxins—food, water, medications and pollution. After many years of tracking what goes into my body and the visual results, there is no doubt in my mind that what we consume affects the skin. Food goes through many more processes with industrial manufacturing than it did even twenty years ago, and we are consuming more packaged foods than ever before. Walking through a grocery store it's easy to see how much of our food is processed. Ninety percent of grocery aisles contain dried, dehydrated packaged foods. For at least ten years, I would watch as my psoriasis went from looking light and pink and flat to deep red, and burning and the only thing that had changed was I went from eating salad one day to eating processed foods on another. After a night out of drinking alcohol, eating pizza, fries and wings, my skin would look much worst for a few days. This went on for so many years that it led me investigate if there was a connection between food and psoriasis. Doctors would always tell me that there is no connection. But, I was confused because there was a marked difference in my skin with the consumption of some foods.

Then, what emerged after increased study of autoimmune disease was the effect of intestines becoming permeable. The leaky gut occurs when the lining of the intestines is damaged and becomes permeable allowing undigested foods, waste material, and bacterial toxins to get into the blood. The intestines are a barrier, which protects the inner tissues from the outside. When leaky gut occurs, the intestines develop tiny holes allowing foreign material to get into the blood, triggering the immune system and contributing to psoriasis outbreaks. So far it's just a theory. There is no cure for psoriasis because currently, there is no research to confirm the connection between leaky gut and psoriasis.

Food, chemicals, pollution, bad bacteria, virtually anything inside of the intestines can get through the intestinal barrier and into the blood with leaky gut, but numerous studies confirm that certain foods and drink, for example alcohol, will increase intestinal permeability whereas tryptophan decreases permeability. This is probably one reason why when I consumed alcohol my psoriasis would spread and get worst within days, but since consuming chicken, turkey and salmon--foods high in tryptophan--my psoriasis healed up completely and remains healed. This is one of the reasons my Psoriasis Detox Diet includes these foods. I believe that long term consumption of the right foods with the right nutrition can help the skin and the body to heal.

People with psoriasis must live with an overactive immune system, being constantly triggered by what they consume which causes it to be overworked and--I believe--leaves us vulnerable to developing worse conditions such as major infections like strep, along with cardiovascular disease, diabetes and cancer. Research confirms that psoriasis is correlated with many of these diseases. One reason is thought to be that when the immune system is constantly in overdrive, it is overworked daily and when a real virus or bacterial infection occurs, the immune system may be in such a weakened state that it cannot attend to more serious problems.

The lining of the intestines covers quite a large surface area in the gut, and its role is not only to keep things out, but it must absorb the right nutrients from food and transport it to the liver. Interesting research reveals that below the intestinal epithelium, there are a variety of immune cells, including B cells, T cells, dendritic cells (DCs), and neutrophils which are all part of the immune system. [10] It therefore makes sense that what we consume could be affecting the immune system directly, especially if the intestinal wall is permeable. This fact means that everything that gets into our digestive tract comes in direct contact with our immune system. Could all the processed food we consume be affecting our immune system for days and weeks, triggering it and leading to more and more psoriasis outbreaks and wreaking havoc on our health? It is yet another reason that led me to cut out all processed foods, particularly those with white flour as part of my Psoriasis Detox Diet. Right away I noticed a reduction in redness and dryness of my psoriasis outbreaks, so I knew I was on the right path.

In addition, to triggering the immune system, when the intestines are affected by leaky gut, the digestive system cannot do its job properly by absorbing proper nutrients. So, we have to be even more careful about what we consume on a daily basis. We have to assist our body as much as possible to alleviate the load we place daily on our intestines, which is why I think liquid smoothies are a necessary addition. I believe that contrary to what the medical community believes, this is the effect of food on our condition. While psoriasis may not be directly related to diet as in an allergic reaction, I believe that what we eat matters if chemicals and particles of processed food, toxins in water and medications are going to get through the intestinal lining and trigger the immune system.

Also, what we eat provides nutrition for the body, but if the digestive system and immune system cannot detect what the food is, it is immediately treated as foreign and must be attacked. For this reason we cannot eat tree bark and get nutrition from it. The body cannot process it. This is true of processed foods. Tree bark or wood may not kill you, but eating it could wear out the digestive system. Why don't we eat paper? It comes from trees, but it has been put through many processes and there is no real nutrition in it. The same is true of processed food, which the food industry passes off as safe.

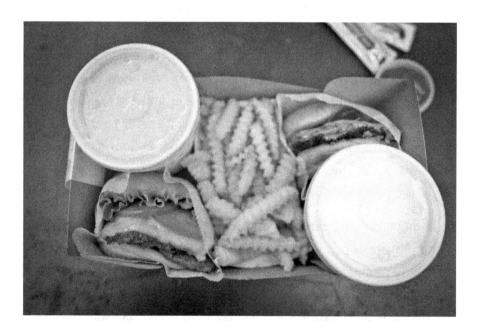

Pizza, pasta, bread, cakes, pies, wraps, cereal and more--all foods placed in a package--have been modified from their natural form. Junk food that we buy form fast food restaurants are the worst as not only are they made from processed ingredients, they contain many hidden thickeners and preservatives.

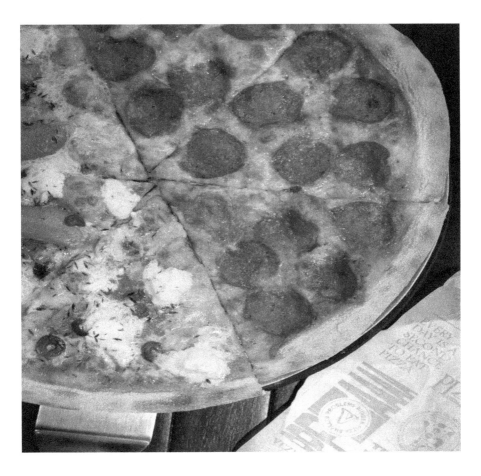

Take one look at the label on packaged foods and it shows a number of unknown chemicals which I often have to research. I believe that if we consume enough of these package foods which contain these chemicals, they may not kill us but, overtime they will probably cause illness and disease.

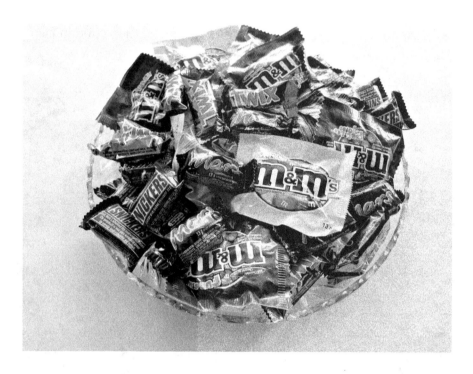

M and M's contain a variety of chocolate and dyes along with dextrin and gum acacia. I researched dextrin and found from Wikipedia that is used in water soluble glues, envelopes, additives in sand casting and printing thickening.

I wondered to myself why do we need this in our food and how does this affect our intestines over time. I figure that an additive used in industrial processes cannot be safe to be consuming long-term in our food. So, I consider people with psoriasis to be fortunate because we get a warning early on with our skin outbreaks. The immune system identifies some foods as toxic and foreign; psoriasis is a warning that the body is becoming overloaded. If these outbreaks did not occur on the skin, would be pay as close attention. In addition, there are so many other diseases which remain undiagnosed until it is too late. Much of the processed food in stores may not affect the average person right away, but for people with psoriasis food sold in packages with preservatives and chemicals have the potential to affect our intestines and it is believed to make leaky gut worst. One of the worst offenders is gluten. It is a protein found in wheat products which directly impacts intestines.

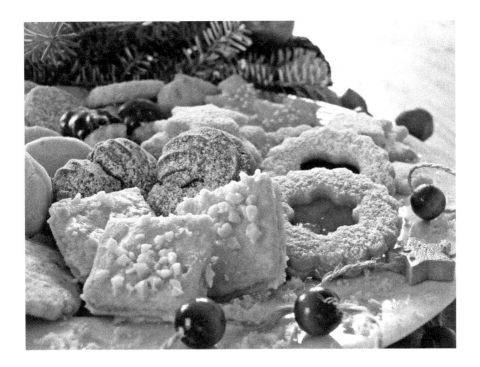

Gluten is one of the worst things for people with psoriasis, and yet, ninety percent of us eat pizza, pasta, bread, cakes, pies, wraps, cereals and crackers week after week. This was one of the first big revelations for me. I cut all processed and packaged goods from my diet, and I immediately saw a huge change in my skin. My psoriasis outbreaks were less red and in a few days they began to flatten and heal. So, removal of all packaged goods became one of the first steps in my clear skin program. For most people these foods are harmless, but I found that my skin never healed completely after even eating the slightest bit of packaged foods. I am so certain that these foods are destroyers of health that I refuse to eat them even today being one hundred percent clear. Processed foods cause another major issue for psoriasis and it is the disruption of bacteria. The digestive system and skin only works when bacteria is balanced.

Numerous studies now show that people with psoriasis and psoriatic disease have major disruptions in bacteria in the gut and the skin. This means that it is even more important for us to replenish with good strains. Probiotics have become front and center for autoimmune and many other conditions. Probiotics are supplements which help to replenish and balance bacteria, but they are even more crucial to psoriasis where the gut is the source of the problem. So I began to realize that it would not matter what I used on my skin, if the digestive system was the source of psoriasis. My question was: If the immune system is in the gut, and what we eat is affecting the gut, how is a steroid cream, which goes on the skin, going to be a long term solution. I understand that doctors have no choice but to prescribe steroid creams as the first standard option for treatment, but it is up to us to know that these creams will not fix leaky gut.

Trying to solve psoriasis with creams is like trying to unclog a stopped up sink by pouring cream onto the drain. It is the same with psoriasis; the skin is only a sign that something very disturbing and problematic is happening deep inside.

The medical system is only able to deal with the signs. Steroid creams and medications like biological, made my outbreaks disappear for a few weeks, but they did nothing to alleviate leaky gut.

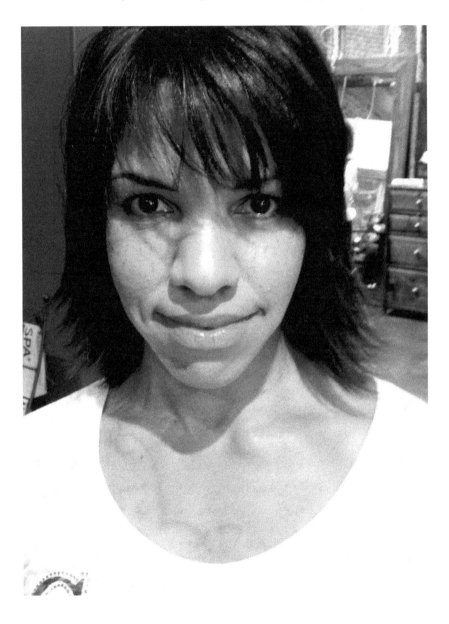

So I witnessed major flare-ups using medications and worst flare-ups when I stopped them. Psoriasis would spread for months--sometimes a year or two--causing me to become desperate and search for the next medication to stop the flare-up. This makes sense because creams on the skin and medications cannot change what is happening in the gut.

So, I searched for natural healing remedies, which I used to address the problems in the digestive system. First, I felt it was important to remove the offenders, inflammatory processed foods which were contributing to leaky gut. Next, if gut bacteria was so important, I felt it was necessary to identify the best probiotic I could find to replenish good bacteria. These two steps alone improved my psoriasis by seventy percent, so I knew I was on the track to healing. This was something I never experienced taking drugs where psoriasis spread to cover most of my body after a few months of application.

When I began to heal from the inside out, I no longer had the side effects I experienced while taking pharmaceutical drugs, and I realize now pharmaceutical drugs merely mask the problem rather than address the source of the problem. Another serious factor to consider is taking all medicines. Research shows that medications like antibiotics disrupt bacteria in the gut, which seems to correlate with the increase of psoriasis. This means every time you have an infection or go in for surgery and take antibiotics, good bacteria is disrupted over and over. Therefore, it is not surprising that people with psoriasis seem to go for years without healing, because so many factors affect the digestive system and contribute to leaky gut which I believe

So I focused on healing my digestive system with a few daily practices. I began to keep a detailed food journal to track every substance going into my body. I used only high-quality supplements made by reputable companies, and I ensured that whatever I put into my digestive system was safe. This became a crucial part of my psoriasis detox program. I removed all foods which were potentially inflammatory or could affect the intestines and replaced them with foods known to be safe and filled with good nutrition.

It makes no sense to fuel the body with processed junk foods, which only disrupt bacteria balance, wear out the digestive system and increase inflammation, triggering the immune system. I was so convinced that processed flour could disrupt digestion, I removed all from my diet and within a couple of weeks I saw a marked improvement in my skin. Until we can put a scope into the digestive system and see what exactly happens with leaky gut, we will never be one hundred percent certain about the relationship between leaky gut and psoriasis, but what we do know is that natural healing of intestines and improving digestive processes leads to a major improvement in psoriasis outbreaks on the skin and even long term clearance.

The major difference between my Psoriasis Detox Diet program and others is that I do not introduce inflammatory or junk foods while there are outbreaks on my skin and the gut is inflamed. Re-introduction only happens weeks after I am completely clear and I believe that this cut down on the potential for Psoriasis to be triggered. In addition, there are other factors which I believe can disrupt gut bacteria and contribute to leaky gut: consuming alcohol, pollution--chemicals in food and drinks as well as stress--all seem to increase inflammation of the intestines. My recourse was to investigate everything that went into my body and remove all destructive substances for as long as it took to clear my skin. I also felt it was important to support the healing process by adding things which are organic and necessary for proper digestive health like: (1) high quality supplements, (2) whole, organic foods with nutrients and fewer chemicals, (3) organic grass-fed meats, which have no hormones and (4) water to flush out all the toxicity that built up over the years. I felt that these practices when combined could restore balance to the intestines and improve digestion.

There is also research focused on the link between a leaky gut and other systemic diseases like celiac disease, Crohn's disease, diabetes, irritable bowel syndrome and many other autoimmune conditions. I learned that modification of lifestyle habits and dietary intake can relieve symptoms in all of these diseases, so it led me to believe that it could help to improve my skin. I was right. Today, after being one hundred percent clear, I know that the key to healing psoriasis is to understand the relationship between psoriasis and the leaky gut syndrome. It makes sense because eighty percent of the immune system lies in the gut, and psoriasis is strongly linked to the immune system. This means that the gut microbiome can be crucial to psoriasis and overall health. We need a working gut that can absorb nutrients but which is still tight enough to prevent bacteria from seeding into the sterile field of the bloodstream.

Many functional and natural doctors have worked on healing the gut to help treat many chronic diseases. While studying nutrition and naturopathy I began to formulate these ideas about natural healing for my psoriasis. Over the years I could see that when I ate certain foods, my skin would react within days. At first I thought it was random, but I followed such a disciplined regime of eating, often consuming the same foods for days. I could clearly see that food had an effect on my skin. I felt that the first step in healing was to remove anything that could contribute to inflammation in the gut. Next, I removed any foods which are known allergens or tend to cause sensitivities. A food sensitivity test can be helpful, but it is not mandatory. Foods, to which we have a sensitivity seem to affect the digestive system, so removing them seems to help calm psoriasis flare-ups.

There is another problem with pharmaceutical medications; they attack the symptoms for a short time but they don't address leaky gut, which is probably why I found they stopped working, and my psoriasis would always get worse. The existence of leaky gut also made me wonder if medications were not making it worse. Antibiotics have been proven to affect gut bacteria, so it would not be surprising if we found that medications were contributing to many of the digestive issues, and therefore making psoriasis worse. I took psoriasis medications for so many years and all I experienced were side effects. There were no changes to my skin, and I only endured the outbreaks getting worse and spreading. What is surprising is that I have not taken antibiotics nor medications in three years, and I have had no skin outbreaks after healing naturally. In fact I have not been ill with a virus or cold in this time either, when previously I would be fighting a cold or flu every couple of weeks. It is possible that I was trapped in a cycle of outbreaks and illness; I would take medications and have more outbreaks leading to worse disruption of my gut. So for a few years, I just focused on healing the intestines and leaky gut.

Natural medicine suggests that to heal leaky gut, the following may be beneficial: probiotics, increase fiber, increase vitamin C, drink at least three liters of water a day and consume bone broth. So, I implemented all of these into my Psoriasis Detox Diet program and my psoriasis healed completely.

# Using Medications VS Natural Healing

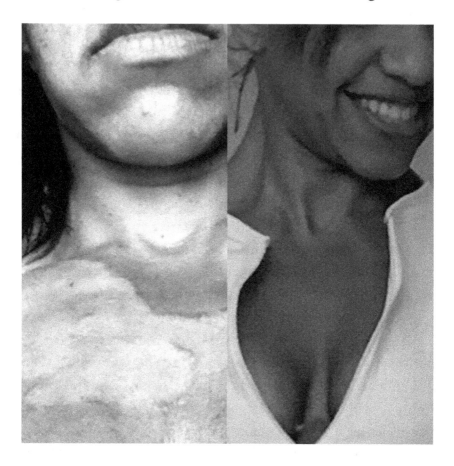

# CHAPTER 4

## *Psoriasis and the Liver*

The liver is a major organ which handles toxins that enter the body. The liver and psoriasis are intimately related, and, as I discovered, many things can negatively impact the liver. Alcohol, smoking, medications, chemicals in food and water, pollution, and synthetic chemicals in creams and lotions can overload the liver. When the liver becomes overloaded it cannot do its job of detoxifying the body, which leaves many of these foreign invaders circulating in the body. The connection between the liver, digestive system, psoriasis and the skin is this: If potential chemicals, food and medications are seeping into the blood through a gut wall, which has become permeable, then the next line of defense is the liver.

We learned previously that people with psoriasis are at risk for fatty liver disease. If the liver is overloaded and already weak, then it is incapable of removing foreign invaders, which eventually trigger the immune system. I came to realize that everything that enters the body must be dealt with by the liver. People with psoriasis face the added challenge of having everything we consume affect the immune system, inflammation and the skin.

I became very concerned that all of the medications and creams I was prescribed and taking for over a decade, could be overloading the liver. This could explain why my skin never healed while I was using these drugs. It made less sense to overload the liver with alcohol and medication and continue this cycle if the result would always be overloading the liver, triggering the immune system and making my skin worst. So, I got fed up, frustrated and decided to remove these pollutants from my body for good. I cut out alcohol, all medications, flour, sugar, dairy and all inorganic meats. I felt I had to remove all inflammatory foods and substances, which could affect the liver. It took several months because I began to remove many foods that I had eaten for years; the detox symptoms were unbearable. You may notice that when you start to remove bad foods and replace them with good foods and lots of water you experience many adverse symptoms like headaches, body aches, fatigue, dizziness and insomnia. I went through this for weeks and later learned that they could result from withdrawal from sugar and caffeine which tend to contribute to experiencing these symptoms. Of course if, these symptoms persist for more than 3 weeks then you must see your doctor. It is one of the reasons I strongly suggest no fasting as the first step in attempting natural healing. Many people swear by fasting, but for those of us who are not used to doing regular fasts, I feel that it is too stringent a step to take as the fist steps in following natural healing.

## What Is A Toxin

Psoriasis has long been linked to toxins building up in the body, getting into the blood and contributing to skin flare-ups. What is a toxin? A toxin is anything that can affect the body's detox organs. Alcohol, smoke from cigarettes and marijuana, pollution, bad bacteria, chemicals, medications, gluten, lectins and harmless food particles are toxins. When these substances enter the blood stream, they trigger the immune system causing a full scale immune system attack, which also overloads the liver and kidneys. So every time you put these things into the body, you can trigger psoriasis. However, the effects may not be seen immediately. It could take a while. Unfortunately one trigger can cause a major flare-up and delay healing for months and years. This is the catch 22. The organs involved in removing toxins are the liver, kidneys, large intestine, lungs and one more important organ, the skin.

Yes, the skin is an organ; it is the main backup organ and it is involved in removal of toxins. Therefore, it is not at all surprising that if psoriasis is linked to toxins, then psoriasis outbreaks occur on the skin. When all of your other organs are overloaded and unable to do their job of ridding the body of toxins, the skin takes over. This occurs in hundreds of complex reactions in the body. So to isolate why psoriasis patches happen is very difficult.

Armed with this information, we need to do the following three things:

- stop toxins from getting into the body.

- alleviate the load on our organs and cleanse the body.

- give the body proper nutrition, so it can do its job and stop affecting the skin.

This was my thinking with dietary changes. I did the following:

- analyzed the food I was eating and substituted processed food with wholesome natural foods.

- increased water which helps cleanse the body.

- added a few supplements for nutrients which could help the body heal.

And it worked. I worked with a basic understanding of the major factors involved in psoriasis. What is interesting is that all of this information about toxicity affecting health is not new. We are warned daily of the effects of toxic food, the importance of eating organic food free of pesticides and hormones. I realized that every person with psoriasis has to take extremely good care to detox their organs, because it is key to clearing the skin.

Toxins can also come in the form of things which are supposed to be good for us like medications. The reason medications can be toxic to the body is because they cause many side-effects. When you take medications, you suffer side-effects, and then you need more medications. This sets us up for another vicious cycle. A good example is when we take psoriasis drugs, which suppress the immune system; we get ill and have to take antibiotics which then seem to cause a worse flare-up of psoriasis, particularly guttate. This has been my experience for many years. It's just fighting a constant vicious cycle of medication, side-effects, more medications, more outbreaks and it is non-stop.

When the liver is overloaded, toxins can build up in the body making it very difficult to remove them. Smoke is a great example of this. When pollutants from smoke enter the body, it is very likely that they will build up in the lungs and blood vessels causing long-term damage. I believe this is just one of the reasons smoking makes psoriasis worse and contributes to the development of other diseases. I kew smoke was a major trigger particularly when, at one time, I was healing using natural remedies and regularly came into contact with second hand smoke and I watched my skin go from being 70% clear to 90% covered with outbreaks in a very short period of time. Unfortunately, vaping and smoking cannabis seems to also affect the skin, so I caution anyone who is smoking and has Psoriasis. It makes sense Smoke which is an unnatural substance goes into the lungs and gets directly into the blood immediately overloading the liver which has to detoxify the body.

When the liver can no longer handle the toxic load, the body is forced to utilize the skin for detoxification, so not only is the immune system triggered and affecting multiplication of skin cells, but toxins are being pushed out through the skin, which increases inflammation, and I believe it makes psoriasis outbreaks worse. Why else would there be varying levels of redness and pain in psoriasis flare-ups ranging from extreme redness and bleeding to dry and flakey conditions? You can see when inflammation decreases; the skin looks pinker and the outbreaks are less inflamed. I think it has a lot to do with the amount of toxic substances that are passed through the skin tissue.

The body's main goal is to ensure that if toxins enter the body from food and drinks, they are eliminated early enough to prevent damage to the body. After dealing with psoriasis, I witnessed the outbreaks looking red and inflamed when I consumed processed food and drink.

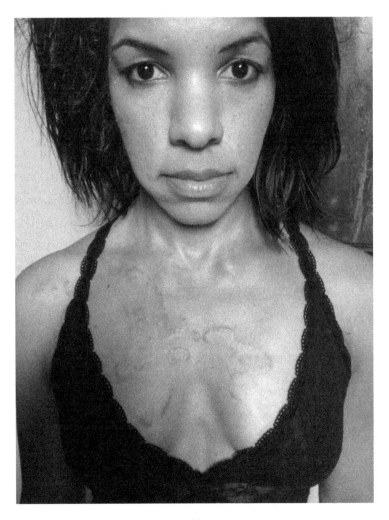

The more I consumed, the worse my skin looked. As soon as I began to reduce the toxic load on my body by following the psoriasis detox plan, my skin began to heal and outbreaks cleared up.

Avoiding toxins is more effective than having to remove them after they build up in the body. I believe that psoriasis is a wakeup call to deal with the toxicity levels of the body and the answer is not to throw more creams and medications at the liver, which is already overworked and cannot handle the current load. Cleansing or detoxification is supposed to happen on a daily basis for all individuals naturally. But, for those who have psoriasis, we need to cleanse the body more frequently which is why I believe that my Psoriasis Detox Diet program helps to support the healing process.

## Psoriasis and Fatty Liver Disease

Fatty liver disease is yet another problem for people with psoriasis. Research shows that it occurs when the liver accumulates too much fat. Alcohol can also contribute to fatty deposits in the liver cells, but there is a second form called non-alcoholic fatty liver disease (NAFLD), which is prevalent in people with psoriasis. Therefore, people with psoriasis have a higher risk of irreversible liver damage and already have an issue with the liver. Add alcohol, medications, processed food, pollution and chemicals in food and water and it is easy to see how the liver can become overloaded. Also, obesity and insulin resistance could lead to fatty liver disease inflammation, so these are also of concern.

Current statistics show that almost forty-seven percent of people with psoriasis tend to develop non-alcoholic fatty liver disease (NAFLD) which I found particularly important because of the hundreds of people I communicated with over two years, At least eighty percent drank alcohol, smoked and were obese, including myself. Once I cut out these things and followed a weight loss program, cleansing the body and the liver, my symptoms vanished. Alcohol and smoking are major factors affecting the liver. Metabolic syndrome is another key contributor to psoriasis as well, because it is related to fatty liver disease. This means that people who have psoriasis and are obese are more likely to also have NAFLD. The potential for fatty liver disease means that it is important to check the liver regularly and maintain it with detox and cleansing.

I found that whole foods eaten in their natural form along with lots of water made a tremendous difference. The ultimate goal is to reduce the toxic burden that the liver gets and by extension relieve the body from having to deal with too many toxins. Some of the best liver foods include onions, garlic turmeric, coconut oil, beet juice, and other green juices. A proper diet has the advantage of reducing the toxins in the body and this helps cleanse the entire system. The body systems are interconnected and related in such a manner that one sluggish part of the system can lead to problems in other systems. The lungs, skin, liver, kidneys, and gut should function well to get the most out of the detox program.

The liver is very resilient and when it is working normally, it can handle the toxins without a problem. Drinking plenty of fresh water helps the liver to filter toxins. Veggies are good for the liver's health because they have vitamins which are part of the machinery required for the breakdown of substances. They metabolize hormones and help the body get more nutrients from the diet without the risk of an increased toxin load. Environmental chemicals and pollution can also affect the body, so it is important to minimize exposure to reduce the load on the detox organs (skin) from the environment. All such chemicals endanger the health of the liver.

# CHAPTER 5

# *Psoriasis and Stress*

S tress is known to be a major factor responsible for the triggering and progression of psoriasis. It's easy to see why. Stress affects many systems in the body including the digestive system. Hans Selye's General Adaptation Syndrome explains why stress is so detrimental to people with psoriasis. GAS describes the stages that the body goes through in stress including alarm, resistance and exhaustion. I believe that one of the reasons it is important to manage stress with psoriasis is that similar to progression of stress which gets worse and worse, so do psoriasis outbreaks. I can recall in childhood when I first got psoriasis, it was a light outbreak on my head. But, the older I got, the worse the outbreaks became. The third stage is the exhaustion stage and I believe that this stage is the most critical for psoriasis as the body is not only in adrenal fatigue but the body will be less capable of healing in the exhaustion stage. The nervous system and psoriasis are related, so I believe depending on which stage of stress we are in, it will determine how fast we can heal psoriasis.

Another factor is the effects of the nervous system on the digestive system. Research shows that when the nervous system is in a sympathetic state, digestion can be affected and even stopped. So when we are stressed it's quite possible that this has a significant impact on digestion which for people with psoriasis, is already compromised. The implication is that when we eat and we are stressed, food is not being digested correctly and may sit around in the digestive system, enabling leaky gut and affecting the balance of bacteria.

I believe the processes which eventually lead to outbreaks include the combination of stress, processed food sitting around in the intestines, chemicals getting through the intestinal wall into the blood and affecting the immune system. It's also accepted that stress and the secretion of adrenaline can cause ulcers in the digestive tract, so it would not be surprising if leaky gut is affected by stress.

Lastly, it is stress that leads to psoriasis, but in some instances psoriasis increases stress. So people with psoriasis become stuck in this pattern of stress triggering psoriasis and more stress making psoriasis worse.

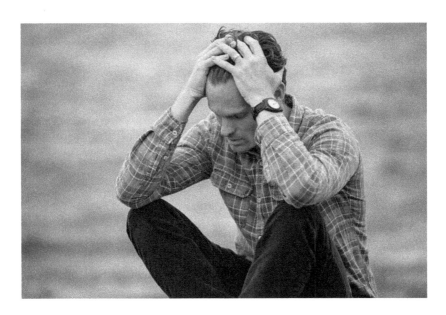

Stress prevents the body from recovering and can contribute to sleep disruptions. When the body does not recover, stress hormones are increased. For people with psoriasis, this becomes a vicious cycle of stress, psoriasis outbreaks, lack of sleep leading to more stress and more flare-ups. Stress increases inflammation in the body, which affects the immune system. So there is a definite connection between psoriasis, stress and the immune system which seems to be at the heart of the triggering of psoriasis. Even people who have autoimmune disease in their family do not seem to be affected by psoriasis unless it is triggered by a stressful event of consuming something that is stressful and harmful to the body. So, if stress is a major factor affecting psoriasis, it is no wonder that medications did not provide a complete solution. While they are effective at shutting down inflammation and the immune system the medications did virtually nothing to help me to manage stress and the stressful events occurring. This could explain why an important part of my Clear Skin program was stress management. I believe that stress management strategies, better sleep and managing other factors which cause stress is the key to managing psoriasis.

## PsychoNeuroimmunology

The connection between psychology, the nervous system and the immune system plus the effects on inflammation is crucial to psoriasis. I was keen to listen when Dr. Mark Hyman and Dr. Leonard Calabrese at a Cleveland clinic discussed the studies, which found connections of our emotions and mental state on inflammation and immune system on Dr. Hyman's podcast called "Farmacy." Researchers have found that behavioral and psychological events can influence the immune system.

Professor Steven Maier, at the University of Colorado said at an APA convention, that the immune system sends signals to the brain which potentially alter neural activity including behavior, thought and mood. This could hold the answer as to why psoriasis is triggered after a strep infection. There seems to be a connection between the immune system, the brain and sickness where it has been found that immune cells create molecules when there is infection, which trigger the brain to alter the systems in the body essentially creating sickness. For people with psoriasis, I believe that it is this "sickness response" which triggers psoriasis. Dr. Maier, in his research was able to inactivate the molecules from affecting the brain and afterward there was no sickness. Further studies show that immune cells activate the vagus nerve through neurotransmitters which send signals to the brain. Once the brain receives these signals, it generates its own Interleuken-1 which affects the immune system more. Dr. Maier has confirmed that stress does the same thing, but it begins in the brain. It suggests that psychological stress can cause illness, and this has been one of the earliest theories about the trigger for psoriasis.

So, what does this mean for the healing psoriasis? It's possible that people with psoriasis, like me, are stressed and this is already affecting the immune system. Add an infection like strep throat and this compounds the effects and leads to increased psoriasis outbreaks. I recall having several bouts of strep infections. In general, psoriasis seems to flare up; then after the strep throat and use of antibiotics, it tends to spread out of control to cover the body. In the case of Guttate, which is the form which seems to be triggered with strep throat, in my experience, it will heal on its own with months of supporting the healing process. Remove the effects of the immune system, as is found in Dr. Maier's world and it calms down and clears up the psoriasis outbreaks. But how does it explain when psoriasis is triggered without strep throat. I believe that other triggers of psoriasis set up a similar pattern. They stress the body in some way and begin the vicious cycle which eventually leads to psoriasis outbreaks. We already know that the other known triggers for psoriasis can also create stress in the body including lack of sleep, alcohol consumption and of course chemicals and processed food. Dr. Maier confirms that he was able to induce a stress response by isolating animals and causing them to become stressed, so it is possible that the mental state, along with the triggers, are crucial pieces of the puzzle. Many people with psoriasis report a stressful event, being stressed, angry or suffering from anxiety, heartache or loss preceded their skin outbreaks. However, there is no doubt that a poor diet, alcohol, pollution and even food sensitivities play a major role along with stress in triggering psoriasis and making skin outbreaks worst.

# CHAPTER 6

# *Common Treatments For Psoriasis*

Currently several drugs are available. Here is my experience with using them.

## Topical Steroids

Medicated and pharmaceutical ointments and creams generally have steroids. These are corticosteroids. These are fast acting and tend to make the skin look better within days, but long term, they cause side effects and often when I stopped, psoriasis spread to cover my body for at least six to eight months. Newer topical therapies include vitamin D creams.

## Shampoos and Oils

A variety of medicated shampoos and oils are available for the hair and scalp. They help with flaking and calm down some of the redness, but I found that after using medicated shampoos--especially those with steroids--the psoriasis spread to different areas of my body.

## Light Therapy

Medically supervised light therapy using UVB is one of the most common and effective methods. The only issue with this treatment is the time it requires. It requires usually three times a week for about thirty sessions. Today, there are home units available which have apps attached so you and your doctor can monitor treatments.

## Systemic Treatment

These are biological medications which affect the immune system. The main purpose of these drugs is to suppress the immune system and to stop the cycle of the immune system being in overdrive and causing the outbreaks on the skin. I tried these drugs for many years, but there was always a problem. Long-term none worked and I had to switch every few months. They are also very expensive and never cleared my skin one hundred percent. They also have horrendous side effects.

## Herbal Medicines

Herbal medicines are often sold online or in health food stores. While some herbs have been found to be beneficial, the majority of what is sold online is suspect. Many are sold by people who have no credentials or training and it is a very unregulated industry. There is no regulating body for herbs, so there is no way to know for sure what is in these products. My personal suggestion after years of trying many of these products is to source highly qualified naturopaths and functional doctors who can show certifications. Many herbal remedies now have hidden steroids which cause symptoms to worsen and will make it much harder to heal psoriasis.

# CHAPTER 7

# Transitioning To Natural Healing

O ne of the challenges I faced was in the period between getting off all medications and following natural healing. I discovered it was one thing to take medications, and it's quite another thing to get off them, because when I cut off both biologics and steroid creams, my psoriasis flared up and spread out of control for many months.

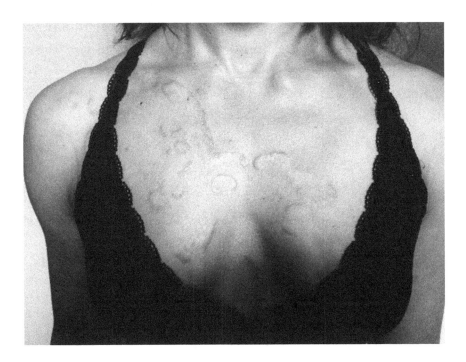

The National Psoriasis Foundation calls this rebounding and it is explained that during the period when you get off medications the skin gets worst before it gets better. I tried to transition to natural healing, but when I stopped medications, my skin flared up so badly that doctors forced me to stop the spread by getting back on more medications. So, essentially I was stuck in a trap familiar to many people with psoriasis. Using medications, skin clears up, get off medications and psoriasis spreads out of control leading to use of more medications. I finally got myself out of this trap when I learned that there are steps to be taken when transitioning from drugs to natural healing. In my experience, steroid creams and psoriasis medications have a withdrawal period of six months to two years or longer, depending on the length of time and the amount of the drug in the body. Over twenty years, I have been in this withdrawal period several times, even being hospitalized on a couple of occasions. So, I strongly recommend that you discuss transitioning off all medications with your doctor and start cleansing and detoxing the body at least one to two months before eliminating medications. Steroid creams in particular must be tapered off slowly.

## Getting off Steroid Creams

Steroid creams caused me to have the worst flare-ups. They worked short term for the first few weeks to clear up the psoriasis, but after this, my psoriasis would always slowly begin to spread. Then when I stopped the cream completely, it spread out of control for months

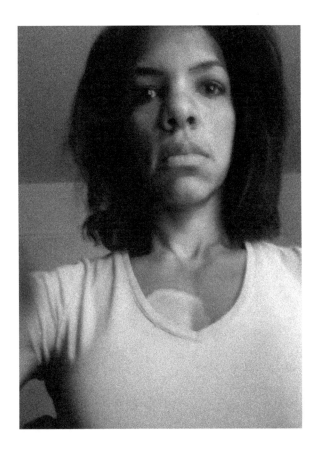

## Using Steroid Creams

I later learned that I should never eliminate steroid medications completely; it was important to reduce them slowly. I did this by cutting the cream down to once a week for about 4 weeks, then once every 2 weeks for another 2 rounds then once every 3 weeks for another 2 weeks then stopped. Never stop steroid creams completely. I did this one a number of occasions and Psoriasis spread out of control and turned to a dangerous form called Erythrodermic which are patches of red inflamed skin. When this happened doctors have no choice but to prescribe medications to prevent infection. It is very important you try to avoid having this happen, but if it does, you must seek medical attention immediately.

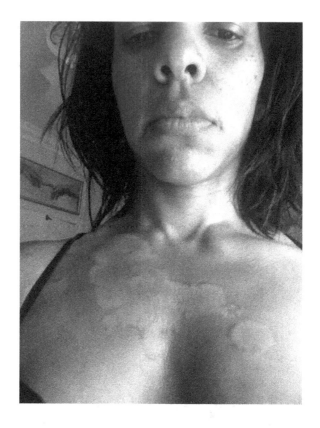

After years of trial and error and discussions with my doctor, I found that the best way to try to transition off of steroids was to continue using it once a week while following my psoriasis detox diet program, for at least 5 or 6 weeks, then start to slowly cut that down over the next few weeks until I finally could stop. This was a significant turning point in helping me to fully transition to natural without the constant flare ups which would result from trying to stop steroid creams. Also, please note that what I did not know at the time is the number of over the counter creams sold on the internet and Ayurveda medicines which have hidden steroids. I have personally had my skin flare out of control with a cream that I did not know contain steroids. So, my suggestion is to be very careful and consult your doctor on everything you are using on your skin that you purchase online or over the counter. Once I could control the flare ups and follow my detox diet program I was able to clear completely.

Previously when I cut the steroids completely, cold turkey, my skin flare up would last months to years which makes it much harder to clear the skin long-term. I found I had to drink a gallon of water a day, and follow my strict diet before I would see any changes to my skin. This is also true of steroids in pill form which have been found to give even worst of a flare up. So take caution and consult your doctor before making the decision to cut steroids out.

## Completely Clear Using My Detox Diet Program

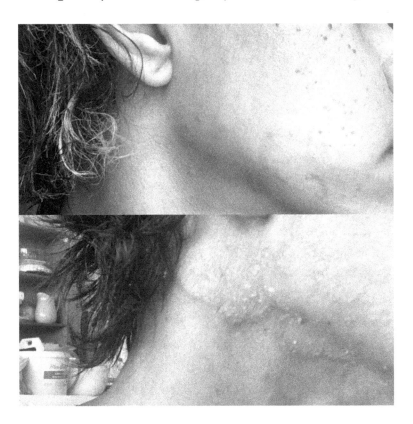

## Getting off Psoriasis Medications

It was an extremely important step when I decided to stop medications. First, I consulted with my doctor to get approval, and then I began trying to eliminate the medications. Previously I would cut the medications and my psoriasis always flared up for months before it got better. I would, of course, panic at the sight of my skin getting worse, but eventually after having this occur many times, I realized it was part of the process. I decided to change this by first, starting with gentle cleansing of the body before cutting the medications. I began this process by drinking three to four liters of water, then I followed the psoriasis detox for at least three weeks before I cut the medications. Then, once I cut the medications, I chose to cut them down slowly, reducing the amounts while I continued following the strict diet until my skin improved. No matter what happens, I suggest to continue to support the healing process with diet, water, sleep and stress management. What I noticed was my skin did get worst before it got better, especially in the beginning stages of the detox. But, long term, there were no scars and my skin cleared completely.

## Cutting Out Smoking and Alcohol

Factors which affect the withdrawal process are consuming alcohol and smoking cigarettes, cannabis, vaping or e-cigarettes. It is important to stop these right away. There will be a period of 3 to 4 weeks after you stop when the skin gets worst before it gets better. But, what I experienced was, after I persist with the following dietary changes and detox, my skin cleared up completely. Alcohol affects the liver and so does toxic chemicals in smoke. So, it was no surprise that both of these made withdrawal periods worst and I found they prevent the healing of my skin. I have personally experienced the agony of cutting out alcohol and smoking and watching my skin get worse fast. I also experienced psoriasis spreading for months before it got better. So, when I finally tried to clear my skin permanently, I found it was important to slowly cut alcohol and smoking.

First I cut all smoking, vaping, weed, etc. I found smoking to be the number one factor which prevents the healing of psoriasis and made it 100 times worse very fast. So when I cut smoking, I cut it out, and then gave it three weeks before any healing began. During this period I recommend drinking three to four liters of water a day. I found that if I did not hit that level each day, nothing happened. Next, I cut out all alcohol. Since evidence of a link between psoriasis and the liver exists, it made sense to me that eliminating alcohol was extremely important to clearing psoriasis. My psoriasis never cleared up completely until I cut alcohol out completely for at least four weeks or longer. So it is necessary to recognize that eliminating alcohol and smoking is not enough. It is important to support the healing process and give it time to heal. What goes in must come out. So putting toxins into the body like smoking and alcohol always results in a period of time, during which it is necessary to cleanse the body. This is where water, dietary changes and stress management help to support the healing process and allow the skin to heal.

## Improve sleep patterns

Another factor which affects withdrawal period and healing is lack of sleep. Insomnia is a detriment. It is only during sleep that the body can heal. So, for people with Psoriasis a lack of sleep can lead to lack of healing. It is important that when you are going through the withdrawal period and trying to heal the skin, you must ensure you get deep sleep preferably between 930PM and 6AM. I was always fascinated by the schedule of athletes. Most never sleep later than 10PM. Why ? Because recovery and sleep have very heavy influence from the sun cycle which affects our own cortisol cycle. So essentially recovery of the body occurs during deep sleep during more hours before midnight. As soon as I improved my sleep, I saw massive changes in my skin. I began by going into bed at 9PM and reading. This helped me to wind down and fall asleep naturally. Electronic devices tend to affect sleep so it is recommended you not even sleep close to your computer, TV or phone. Keep them out of your bedroom. A warm bath at night also helps to relax the body before sleep.

## Increase Daily Water Intake

Since the whole point of following natural remedies is to cleanse the body and get rid of all the toxic buildup which may have overloaded the liver and kidneys and contributing to triggering the immune system, I found it was extremely important to ensure I drank 15 glasses of water a day. This may seem excessive, but I found when I hit this amount, my haling sped up and my skin healed much faster. Water helps to get nutrients into the cells and toxic waste out. It also helped to keep me regular. I feel that increased circulation and optimal colon function is key to helping the body to heal Psoriasis outbreaks. Within a few weeks of drinking 15 glasses of water I began to notice massive changes in my skin. I credit the complete healing of my Psoriasis partially to drinking this much water that I still continue to do this today, even while I am clear.

## Exercise

Exercise in the form of light cardio, weight training, walking, jogging and spin classes seemed to really help the healing of my skin.

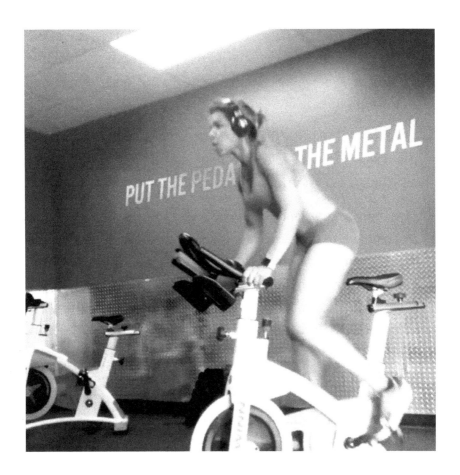

While there is no direct evidence that links exercise with Psoriasis, I felt that exercise since is important for health - it increases circulation, moves the lymphatic system which is related to the immune system, keeps organs strong and helps with stress management I felt that it could help Psoriasis. And it did. I credit doing light exercise 3 times a week with speeding up the healing process, as I saw a tremendous difference in my skin when I added it in. I still exercise today and I feel it has helped with keeping my skin clear for years. Psoriasis is also linked to obesity. National Psoriasis Foundation reported on their website that researchers in Utah found that a great percentage of people developed Psoriatic Arthritis, and Psoriasis were obese and those who are obese later on have a greater risk of developing it earlier than those at a healthy weight. So, I focused on maintaining my weight through the use of exercise.

Just increasing something that the body needs desperately accelerated the healing of Psoriasis. I knew this to be so fundamental, even though I am clear years later, I drink this much water each day without fail.

After speaking to thousands of people with Psoriasis I know that this is one crucial piece of the puzzle as 95% did not consume enough water. Most reported they consumed less than 1 liter. The results made sense. The more toxic matter buildup that the body has to deal with, the more overloaded the detox organs the more the skin ahs to get involved to protect the body as the back up detox organ. The less water we consume the less nutrients can get into the cells to begin the healing process. Engineering had taught me Occam's razor- the simplest solution is often the correct one. What made more sense – taking 10 bottles of supplements trying to heal the body ? or allowing the body's own healing ability to be supercharged with some help. I found that the latter was true. Less is more when it came to healing Psoriasis and clearing the skin.

The second most important part of nutrition is getting actual nutrition into cells and the body to heal. We would not put sugar into the gas tank of our car to make it run, so why do we put it into our bodies. I began to analyze what was the exact nutrition going into my body and I realized, in horror that 80% of it breaks down to sugar. Sugar is not a nutrient known for healing the skin, so why are we eating so much of it. I made a drastic change with the introduction of the green smoothie. Vegetables are packed with nutrition, so I knew that the more I put into my body the better it would be.

Green smoothies serve two purposes – the first is it is liquid nutrition. Easy on the digestive system so it gives our gut a break. I figured if the source of my Psoriasis could be related to the digestive system and an overloaded liver then perhaps giving these systems a mini vacation, may not be a bad idea. Nature takes its time. A seed planted takes weeks to grow and nature allows it to take its course and pretty soon something amazing develops. I adopt this very philosophy with my approach to natural healing. The body needs time to heal at its own pace. Just as we give the seed some water and nutrients from the soil, I figured the same is true of our skin. The second reason green smoothies are so beneficial is that Psoriasis responds to alkalinity. So green smoothies, naturally alkalize the body. I focused on having one in the morning and one at night, so my body remains alkali for most of the 24 hours in a day. This simple step was the second most crucial step to healing my skin. I was absolutely convinced that just focusing on these two steps for a few weeks would dramatically change my skin. I was right. My psoriasis began to clear faster than it ever did before.

The third step to natural healing is providing the nutrients which can support healing but which are difficult to get in food. The average diet consist of cereal or eggs in morning, pizza, pasta sandwiches for lunch and rice with meat for dinner. If we look at the content of these foods what we find is a lot of carbs and sugar and very few actual vitamins, minerals and enzymes. So when our bodies require vit D, essential fatty acids, vit C, vit A, vit B all to heal the skin and it is not present in the foods we are eating, no healing can happen. I believe this is one of the big reasons why Psoriasis does not heal for 90% of the population. The body requires proper nutrition every single day to heal. So, the best way to ensure we provide these essential nutrients to eat whole foods which have lots of vitamins and minerals and to add supplements to our regimen. People scoff at supplements but I found there are a number of good ones which when taken daily can, speed up the healing process.

## The Healing Process

Most functional doctors will agree that psoriasis is not a skin disease. It begins in the gut. If what we are consuming affects the gut which triggers the immune system eventually affecting the skin, then natural healing begins with removing the foods and drink which is potentially triggering the immune system. The question is why does this happen for people with Psoriasis and not for others. I believe that the auto-immune gene predisposes us to a more sensitive system. It is a similar reason as to why some people can eat large amount of foods and never gain weight, similarly, people can consume large amounts of processed junk food and nothing happens. For people with Psoriasis, processed junk food is viewed as a toxin and foreign invader by the body. We know this because when I replaced bad foods with good nutrient filled whole foods there is a dramatic change in the appearance of the skin. I feel that in natural healing the three biggest factors to address are gluten sensitivity, yeast overgrowth and heavy metal poisons. I believe that all 3 are toxic to the body and will cause Psoriasis to continue to breakout and flare up long-term. When we remove gluten from the body and cleanse the body it begins to reduce inflammation. Cleansing seems to help the regeneration of the liver. My skin was visibly, less red and outbreaks began to fade away. The research on fatty liver disease and psoriasis in The Journal of Dermatology show that people with psoriasis are more likely to have fatty liver disease which means we may have a liver which is already underperforming and incapable of handling the added stress and toxic load from toxicity we encounter in food, drink, medications, pollution, alcohol and smoking. People with Psoriasis not only battle an immune system in overdrive, but now it seems that the liver is a major issue as well. So, more than ever, I realized I needed to be extremely careful about what I was allowing into my body.

The digestive system has an extremely important role in psoriasis as this is where everything we consume is processed and it is the connection of the outside environment with the inner. The digestive system also contains one of the biggest parts of the immune system which is found in the set of cells called Peyers Patches. So it is here that what we consume, food, drink and bacteria can have a direct impact on the immune system. If we all are honest with ourselves, every person with psoriasis has eaten food which is not healthy and which can be classified as junk food. The danger is that other people can get away with eating large amounts of junk food; they can gain weight, become obese and take lots of drugs each day. People with psoriasis, however, seem to have a low tolerance level for junk food because everything we consume comes into contact with the Immune system. Could it be the overload of chemicals in food, pollution, toxins along with bacteria which is setting off the immune system. It makes sense that the body could mistake these things for major threats to the body. It's not surprising that the body would be so intelligent to know that a build of toxins would be a threat to the health of the body. It is no secret that the body will store toxins in fat to prevent them circulating in the blood causing harm to our organs, so it would not be impossible for, in the case of Psoriasis, the body triggers the skin as the secondary detox organ to try to deal with the toxic overload. So, in the case of people with Psoriasis, the immune system is being triggered over and over, leading to an increase in inflammation and eventually to affecting the skin. Some people with psoriasis cannot withstand one day of drinking alcohol, eating food containing gluten nor, fried foods. From my experience with psoriasis, what we eat greatly contributes to outbreaks of patches on the skin, and this continues to spread with even the slightest amount of food which are problematic. These foods may not show up on an allergy test because psoriasis is not an allergy. The root of psoriasis is not histamine, released triggering an allergic reaction. It has much more to do with the digestive system, leaky gut and an overloaded liver. I feel that this is where most people trying to follow the natural path go wrong. After listening and speaking to hundreds of people who claimed to have changed their diets, with no effect on psoriasis patches, I realized that they made one major mistake.

Psoriasis will not respond to cutting out one or two foods and hoping that the skin heals. The approach to healing has to be more holistic. I created my Psoriasis Detox Diet program to address all this things which must be done daily over a period of several weeks to help to support the healing process. This is very similar to the autoimmune protocol which was largely dismissed until ten years ago when actual research revealed that it was an acceptable way to control autoimmune disease. Doctors support the autoimmune protocol and my program follows many similar principles.

Inflammation is at the source of inflammatory diseases and reducing inflammation is the cornerstone of natural healing. Psoriasis warriors try hundreds of popular diets but many of these many diets simply do not remove inflammation. Just because a diet may help with weight loss doesn't mean it will heal the skin. For this reason, many people report no benefit, with diets for psoriasis. My Psoriasis Detox Diet program is based on the principles of removing the foods which cause inflammation, decreasing inflammation seems to calm down the immune system and allows the skin to heal naturally. I feel that the key is to reduce inflammation while providing the necessary nutrients to help the skin to heal, keeping the alkalinity levels high. These are all necessary for healing Psoriasis.

The main difference between my Psoriasis Detox Diet program and the Autoimmune protocol for natural healing, is the removal of foods for six to eight weeks or longer until the skin cleared with no re-introduction. I found that unlike Autoimmune Protocol that allows re-introduction pretty fast, I found that re-introduction of foods before the skin heals triggered my psoriasis over and over. I was able to clear my skin completely remaining off all these foods for 6 to 8 weeks, and remain clear, to this day, 3 years later. For long term success, I feel it is necessary to address all of the issues together, remove the foods irritating the intestines, improve elimination and colon health, detox the body to lessen the burden on the liver and the kidneys, hydrate the body so nutrients can circulate and toxins can be removed and move the body so you keep the lymphatic system strong since this affects the immune system. Lastly, improve sleep so the body can recover. My program not only cleared my skin completely, it also helped thousands of people who followed it and achieved such phenomenal results. My Instagram -@Skinfighters has lots of great examples of transformation stories from people who cleared their skin completely following nothing but natural healing.

# CHAPTER 8

# *Natural Healing*

After fifteen years of constantly battling flare-ups and trying dozens of medications, creams, ointments, herbal medicines and more, I made the decision to follow natural healing. I was fed up and disillusioned. I had taken medication after medication for years and despite following everything my doctors gave me, my skin was still covered in horrific patches of psoriasis.

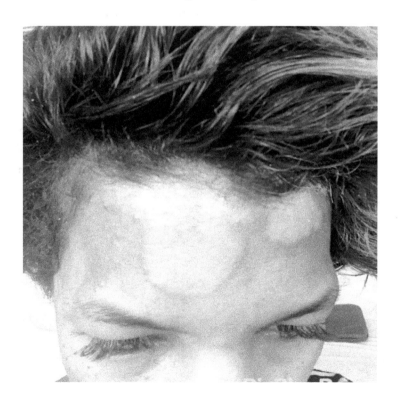

What was worst was the pain from psoriatic arthritis was beginning to prevent normal movement. I would be at school or work, and then all of a sudden I would have an ache in my back or neck that caused everything to seize up and for which I had to lie on the floor to get relief. On a daily basis I would wake up with aches and pains in my shoulder, the back of my knees and my ankles. It was beginning to get out of control. At first, I was skeptical about natural healing. First, it was not accepted by the medical community and most people thought it was hocus pocus. The only reason I turned to natural healing was after consistently trying natural remedies and seeing the results, I had never seen before. After this, I was so convinced, I just began to do everything from taking natural supplements and special diets to baths, steams, teas and more. I had already been involved with fitness for several years, having learned about anatomy, physiology, biology and exercise science in an effort to strengthen my body and improve my health. I also completed 2.5 years study at the Canadian School of Natural Nutrition to study naturopathy, natural nutrition and holistic healing. This education changed my understanding of how to heal the body from the inside out and how nutrition and what we consume impacts health and the skin.

I began my research into all things related to skin diseases, gut health, colon health, the liver and the immune system. I learned that although there were no medical studies to support the success of diet with clearing psoriasis, there was practical evidence popping up every day regarding people who cleared their skin using natural remedies, so I experimented with all things natural. The most important decision I made was to take full responsibility for everything I put into my body. I no longer wanted to treat my body like a garbage can. That's what I had been doing–eating processed fast food. That day, I decided that I would delve deep inside to figure out how food was affecting my skin and make the changes from the inside out.

Until then, I was leaving everything up to my doctors and all the medications, light therapy and creams only worked on the symptoms, so even if I saw a slight change in the skin, it was only temporary. I needed an overhaul. I began to make changes to my diet; I did detoxes, cleanses, and took dozens of supplements. I spent hours dissecting research studies and scientific papers on auto-immune disease, skin diseases and psoriasis during my time at CSNN.

Through my research and study in nutrition and naturopathy, this is how I came to understand the role of food in the psoriasis disease. It is here that I first had lots of information about the theories which had become accepted, that people with psoriasis had "leaky-gut" which caused the intestines to be permeable and allow food particles to get into the blood stream. As soon as I understood this issue, I began to focus on this aspect as I believed this was where it all began. If everything we consume eventually gets into the gut and seeps into intestines floating around in the blood triggering the immune system, then my plan was to stop the foods that could be making leaky gut worst and focus on healing the gut. I spent years trying elimination diets and taking supplements to heal the gut. However, it was not this simple. I would see improvements within weeks of cleaning up my diet, but it would never be 100% clearance. I logged every detail and noted all changes from the different things I consumed. I began to notice that when I consumed certain foods, my psoriasis would be worse. It would be red and spread fast. This happened in 2009. My psoriasis was very mild after trying many cleanses and detoxification diets, but there were still some very small spots. I vacationed in the Caribbean, where I ate more red meat and desserts than usual. And I drank a lot of alcohol. What was shocking was after just three days of that type of eating and drinking, psoriasis patches on my body began to quickly spread. Within two weeks, what started as a couple of spots turned into large patches. That was my first lesson in how diet changes could adversely affect psoriasis, and I knew there was a connection.

Over the next several years I continued to experiment with cleansing and changes in my diet.

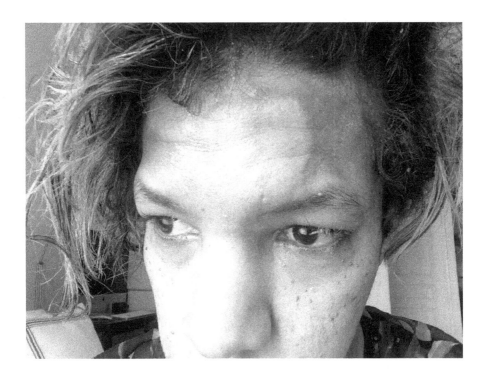

I tried several small detoxes using juicing and vegan diets. While I saw the most improvement from incorporating raw foods into my diet, I still could never get to the point of being 100% clear. I learned that all the processed foods we eat--though they are harmless for most peo-ple--are harmful for people with psoriasis. More and more theories were emerging about how diet affects our bodies, and I gathered that people with psoriasis have problems with the intestines and digestive system. Overgrowth of bacteria, candida, along with processed food, chemicals, drugs and pollution can affect our intestines, leading to developing leaky gut. But, the answer was not to attack everything at once. In our desperation people with psoriasis try all sorts of remedies all at once and only after years of being unsuccessful did I realize that while all of these remedies are helpful, when they are taken together, they seemed to overwhelm the body and prevent my skin from healing completely.

## The First Steps to Natural Healing

One day I decided to change my approach. While dietary changes and supplements were doing a better job improving the look of my skin, it was never clearing 100%. I simplified my approach. I worked on one thing each week until I began to see massive improvements in the outbreaks. The very first step I felt in natural healing was not to limit the number of supplements I was taking and to remove as many as possible. It is normal for people with Psoriasis to want to take every supplement which has ben shown to have even the slightest effect on the skin. We tend to take turmeric, sarsaparilla, vit c, zinc, apple cider vinegar and probiotics all at the same time. While these supplements have been show to have some effect, I believe that taking them all at once at the beginning of the detox process actually slowed my healing down.

The first step in my natural healing journey was to remove all supplements and spend two weeks working on drinking 3 liters or more of water a day. Why was this so important? Our body is 60% water. Nutrients get into cells and toxic waste gets out of cells through diffusion which means if we look at the root cause of everything, it is happening at the cellular level. I realized that the most fundamental part of healing is consuming enough water to ensure everything is flowing at the cellular level, while increasing circulation of nutrients throughout the body and helping toxins to leave the body.

We established that the source of psoriasis is in the digestive system, but if toxins, food particles and bacteria are clogging the digestive system, the skin cannot heal. What's worst is that toxins which are overloading the body cannot get out, so I decided to focus on water intake and ensure I drank 15 glasses a day. It was easy to keep count ensure I hit this amount. What I witnessed was nothing short of miraculous. After a few weeks of just doing this one step, I saw a tremendous difference in my skin, health, sleep and overall well-being. Just increasing something that the body needs desperately accelerated the healing of psoriasis. I considered this step to be so fundamental that even though I am clear years later, I drink this much water each day without fail. After speaking to thousands of people with psoriasis I know that this is one crucial piece of the puzzle as 95% did not consume enough water. Most reported they consumed less than 1 liter. The results made sense. The more overloaded the detox organs became the more the skin had to get involved to protect the body as the backup detox organ. The less water we consume the less nutrients can get into the cells to begin the healing process. Engineering had taught me the Occam's razor principle—the simplest solution is often the correct one. What made sense? Taking ten bottles of supplements to heal the body or allowing the body's own healing ability to be supercharged with some help. I found that the latter was true. Less is more when it comes to healing psoriasis and clearing the skin.

## Skin Begins to Heal With Natural Remedies

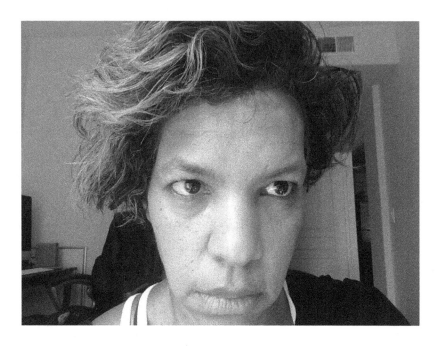

The second most important part is getting nutrition into cells and the body to heal. We would not put sugar into the gas tank of our car to make it run, so why do we put it in our bodies. I began to analyze what was the exact nutrition going into my body and I realized in horror that 80% of it breaks down to sugar. Sugar is not a nutrient known for healing the skin, so why are we eating so much of it? I made a drastic change with the introduction of the green smoothie. Vegetables are packed with nutrition, so I knew that the more I put into my body the better it would be. Green smoothies serve two purposes—the first is it is liquid nutrition. It is easy on the digestive system so it gives our gut a break. I figured if the source of my psoriasis could be related to the digestive system and an overloaded liver, then perhaps giving these systems a mini vacation may not be a bad idea.

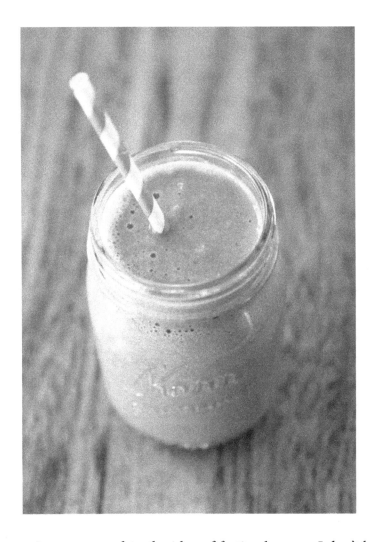

However, I was opposed to the idea of fasting because I don't believe in starving the body. Though it could be helpful later on, I feel that it was too drastic a step to take on at the introduction of natural healing. Nature takes its time. A seed planted takes weeks to grow and nature allows it to take its course and pretty soon something amazing develops. I adopt this very philosophy with my approach to natural healing. The body needs time to heal at its own pace. Just as we give the seed some water and nutrients from the soil, I figured the same is true of our skin. The second reason green smoothies are so beneficial is that psoriasis responds to alkalinity and green smoothies naturally alkalize the body. I focused on having one in the morning and one at night, so my body remains alkali for most of the twenty-four hours in a day. This simple step was the second most crucial step to healing my skin. I was absolutely convinced that just focusing on these two steps for a few weeks would dramatically change my skin. I was right. My psoriasis began to clear faster than ever before.

The third step to natural healing is providing the nutrients which can support healing but which are difficult to get in food. The average diet consists of cereal or eggs in morning, pizza, pasta sandwiches for lunch and rice with meat for dinner. If we look at the content of these foods, what we find is a lot of carbs and sugar and very few actual vitamins, minerals and enzymes. So I cut out most processed and junk foods at this point. So when our bodies require vitamin D, essential fatty acids, vitamin C, vitamin A, vitamin B to heal the skin and it is not present in the foods we are eating, no healing can happen. I believe this is one of the big reasons why psoriasis does not heal for 90% of the population. The body requires proper nutrition every day and consumption of processed fast food slowed down the healing process. I saw tremendous changes in my skin when I removed the following foods from my diet.

# Foods To Be Avoided

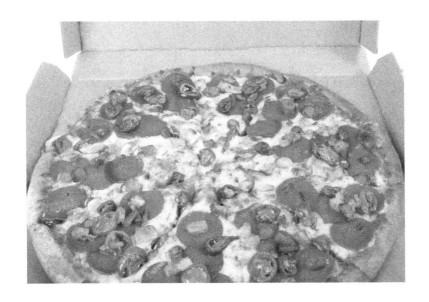

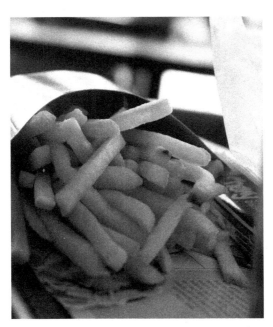

Fast Foods have preservatives and chemicals in it which can increase inflammation and make the skin worst.

## Foods To Be Avoided Cont'd

It is also important to cut out all foods with nitrates like cold cuts and dairy, like milk and cheese, as these also increase inflammation.

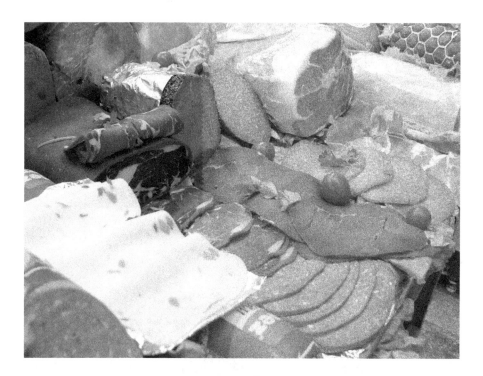

The best way to ensure we provide these essential nutrients is to eat whole foods which have lots of vitamins and minerals and to add supplements to our regimen. Some people scoff at supplements, but I found that a number of good ones if taken daily can speed up the healing process.

## The Healing Process

Most functional doctors agree that psoriasis is not a skin disease. It begins in the gut. What we consume affects the gut which triggers the immune system and eventually affects the skin. Natural healing begins with removing the foods and drinks which are triggering the immune system. The question is why does this happen for people with psoriasis and not for others. I believe that the autoimmune gene predisposes us to have a more sensitive system. It is similar to why some people can eat large amounts of foods and never gain weight; similarly, people can consume large amounts of processed junk food and nothing happens to them.

For people with psoriasis, processed junk food is viewed as toxic and treated as a foreign invader by the body. When I replace bad foods with good-nutrient-filled whole foods, there is a dramatic change in the appearance of my skin and my body. Toxic food is inflammatory so it makes sense that overloading the body with junk food increases inflammation which is at the source of Psoriasis. I feel that in natural healing the three biggest factors to address are gluten sensitivity, yeast overgrowth and heavy metal poisons. I believe that all three are toxic to the body and will cause psoriasis to continue long-term to break out and flare up. When we remove gluten from the body and cleanse the body, it begins to reduce inflammation. Cleansing seems to help the regeneration of the liver. My skin was visibly less red and outbreaks began to fade very quickly after removing processed food form my diet. The research on fatty liver disease and psoriasis in *The Journal of Dermatology* show that people with psoriasis are more likely to have fatty liver disease, which means we may have a liver which is already underperforming and incapable of handling the added stress and toxic load from toxicity we encounter in food, drink, medications, pollution, alcohol and smoking.

People with psoriasis not only battle an immune system in overdrive, but now it seems that the liver is a major issue as well. So, more than ever, I realized I needed to be extremely careful about what I was allowing into my body. The digestive system has an extremely important role in psoriasis as this is where everything we consume, is processed and it is the connection of the outside environment with the inner body. The digestive system also contains one of the biggest parts of the immune system, which is found in the set of cells called Peyers Patches. So that what we consume--food, drink and bacteria--can have a direct impact on the immune system. If we all are honest with ourselves, every person with psoriasis has eaten food which is not healthy and which can be classified as junk food. The danger is that other people can get away with eating large amounts of junk food; they can gain weight, become obese and take lots of drugs each day. People with psoriasis, however, seem to have a low tolerance for junk food because everything we consume comes into contact with the immune system. Could it be the overload of chemicals in food, pollution, toxins along with bacteria which is setting off the immune system. It makes sense that the body could mistake these things for major threats to the body. It's not surprising that the body would be so intelligent to know that a buildup of toxins would be a threat to the body's health. It is no secret that the body will store toxins in fat to prevent their circulating in the blood and causing harm to our organs. So it is possible in the case of psoriasis, for the body to trigger the skin as the secondary detox organ to deal with the toxic overload, once the liver becomes beaten down with the daily task of dealing with this overload.

In the case of people with psoriasis, the immune system is being triggered over and over, leading to an increase in inflammation and eventually to affecting the skin. Some people with psoriasis cannot withstand one day of drinking alcohol, eating food containing gluten, nor fried foods. From my experience with psoriasis, what we eat greatly contributes to outbreaks of patches on the skin, and this continues to spread with even the slightest amount of problematic food. These foods may not show up on an allergy test because psoriasis is not an allergy. The root of psoriasis is not histamine, released triggering an allergic reaction. It has much more to do with the digestive system, leaky gut and an overloaded liver. I feel this is where most people go wrong when trying to follow the natural path. After listening and speaking to hundreds of people who claimed to have changed their diets, with no effect on psoriasis patches, I realized that they made one major mistake. Psoriasis will not respond to cutting out one or two foods and hoping that the skin heals. The approach to healing has to be more holistic. I created my Psoriasis Detox Diet program to address all these things, which must be done daily over a period of several weeks to support the healing process. This is very similar to the autoimmune protocol which was largely dismissed until ten years ago when actual research revealed that it was an acceptable way to control autoimmune disease. Even doctors support the autoimmune protocol and my program follows many similar principles.

Inflammation is at the source of inflammatory diseases and reducing inflammation is the cornerstone of natural healing. Psoriasis warriors try hundreds of popular diets, but many of these many diets simply do not remove inflammation. Just because a diet may help with weight loss doesn't mean it will heal the skin. For this reason, many people report no benefit with diets for psoriasis. My Psoriasis Detox Diet program is more than a diet. It's based on the principles of removing the foods which cause inflammation; decreasing inflammation seems to calm the immune system and allows the skin to heal naturally. I feel that the key is to reduce inflammation while providing the necessary nutrients to help the skin heal. It is important to keep the alkalinity levels high as well as hydration. These are all necessary for healing psoriasis.

The main difference between my detox diet program and the Autoimmune protocol (AIP) for natural healing, is the removal of foods for six to eight weeks or longer until the skin clears with no re-introduction. Unlike the Autoimmune Protocol that allows re-introduction pretty fast, I found that re-introduction of foods before the skin heals triggered my psoriasis over and over. I was able to clear my skin completely remaining off all these foods for 6 to 8 weeks, minimum and I remain clear, to this day, 4 years later. For long term success, I feel it is necessary to address all of the issues together, remove the foods irritating the intestines, improve elimination and colon health, detox the body to lessen the burden on the liver and the kidneys, hydrate the body so nutrients can circulate and toxins can be removed, and move the body so you keep the lymphatic system strong since this affects the immune system. Lastly, improve sleep so the body can recover. My Clear Skin program not only cleared my skin completely; it also helped thousands of people who followed it and achieved such phenomenal results.

My Instagram -Skinfighters has lots of great examples of transformation stories from people who cleared their skin completely following nothing but natural healing and my Psoriasis Detox Diet program.

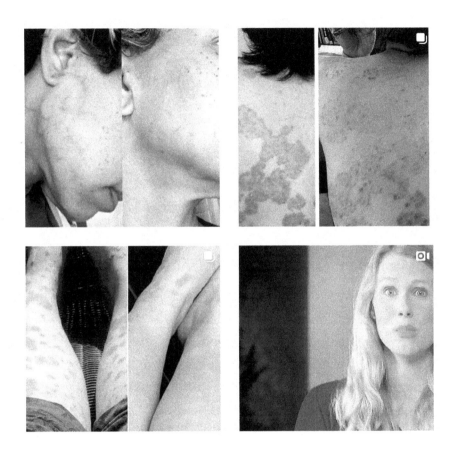

# CHAPTER 9

# Other Remedies for Natural Psoriasis Healing

T here are many other daily practices and remedies we can add to support the healing of psoriasis. Healing from the inside out requires a holistic approach. So adding additional healing remedies can speed up clearing of the skin

## Sun Exposure (Ten to Fifteen Minutes is Recommended)

The sun is extremely important for psoriasis. It provides UVB rays, which have been found to be beneficial for the stimulation of vitamin D in the body and helps heal the skin. In research done by Harvard Health Dr. Olbricht found that though a vitamin D deficiency doesn't cause psoriasis, it may affect the health of the skin and people with psoriasis have been found to have a vitamin D deficiency. I learned that since many people with psoriasis are deficient in vitamin D, stimulating vitamin D has been shown to help. Indoor tanning beds have been shown to emit UVA rays which can be harmful to the body, so using tanning beds is not advised. Medically supervised narrow band light therapy administered by a doctor has been shown to be the best for light therapy.

Vitamin D has been found to be related to the immune system. When the body is deficient in vitamin D, the immune system is immediately affected. This is probably why we often are more susceptible to colds and flus during winter. I can recall being ill every 3 weeks in winter when I lived in Canada. It's one of the coldest countries in the world and it's very gray with very little sunshine between December and May. It's a long time to have very little vitamin D created from the sun, and I noticed my skin was always markedly worse during the winter. I began the practice of standing outside during winter for 10 minutes allowing the sun to hit my face. Just this simple practice helped my skin to improve dramatically even during the colder months. I still do it today for health even though I am completely clear and remaining clear. During the warmer months, I will try to get out in the sun as much as possible. I found if it is possible it helps to take mini vacations to hot tropical destinations during the winter. December to January is a good time because I found it helped me to get through the extremely long winter periods.

## Fish Oil

Omega-3 fatty acids, commonly found in fish and fish oil supplements, have been shown to reduce inflammation and improve psoriasis. Omega-3 fatty acids, eicosapentaenoic acid (EPA) and docosahexaenoic acid (DHA), reduce symptoms and limit the spread of the inflammatory process. I can recall the moment when I learned that every cell in the body is composed of a layer of fatty acids. I realized that if we want to create healthy new skin cells, we would probably need to ensure we have sufficient fatty acids in the body. Since we get so little, I feel it is necessary to supplement with it. I personally took a source of Omega-3 each day, twice a day, and I believe that it helped my skin heal faster. Essential fatty acids are found in fish like mackerel, salmon and sardines so adding these foods to my diet was important.

## Probiotics

Probiotics are friendly bacteria that can be found in yogurt, fermented foods, and supplements. Experts agree that the right balance of bacteria in the body helps the immune system. Because psoriasis is an autoimmune disease, probiotics may be helpful in managing psoriasis symptoms. A study in the journal *Gut Microbes* suggests that a certain type of probiotics may help regulate certain inflammatory responses in the body that contribute to psoriasis symptoms.

## Aloe Vera

The gel from inside an aloe vera plant is known to help heal skin wounds. It may also help reduce redness, scaling, and inflammation from psoriasis. Aloe should be applied directly to the skin, not taken internally. Anyone using an aloe cream should check the label and choose one that contains at least 0.5 percent aloe. Many health food stores carry aloe creams and gels.

## Apple Cider Vinegar

Apple cider vinegar can be particularly helpful to soothe the itching and burning associated with scalp psoriasis. It contains natural germ-killing properties and can be soothing for the scalp. It should not be applied to broken or cracked skin. For a gentler treatment, the vinegar can be diluted with equal parts water. If it burns when applied, stop using it.

## Moisturizers

Bathing in oatmeal or Epsom salts may help to relieve symptoms of psoriasis. Because itching and flaking can make psoriasis look and feel worse, it is important to keep skin moisturized. The most helpful moisturizers are those with natural ingredients and no harsh chemicals. (Try warm baths with salts or oats.)

Bathing has been shown to help psoriasis. First, it is very relaxing, so it helps with stress management, but it also softens the skin and helps to easily remove the scales which build up with outbreaks.

## Natural Lotions

Psoriasis can result in dry patches all over the body. They can become itchy, cracked and eventually bleed. Moisturizing helps to keep the skin smooth and hydrated. I recommend using creams with natural ingredients since anything placed on the skin can be absorbed into the body.

## Humidify

Dry indoor air is associated with dry skin, which is bad news for psoriasis sufferers. Use a room humidifier to raise the humidity.

## The Best Supplements for Psoriasis

These are just a few of the supplements that I took and felt were important to helping to support the healing process and clear the skin.

**Turmeric** – This is one of the best supplements because not only is in an anti-inflammatory, research has shown that it is effective and that it can affect cytokines, which have a tremendous effect on psoriasis.

**Aloe Vera** – I feel that aloe vera is very soothing and seems to reduce redness, inflammation, and scaling.

**Epsom Salts** – I feel that a bath at night helps with stress relief and soothes burning skin outbreaks. Epsom salt, Dead Sea salt and oats soothes the skin and reduce itching.

**Omega 3 Fatty Acids** – I took this in the form of fish oil and flaxseed oil. It calms inflammation, redness and itching and I believe it helped to heal the skin.

**Probiotics** – I felt this was mandatory and I used a liquid one. Psoriasis is related to bacteria imbalances and probiotics replenish good bacteria.

**D3** – Most people with psoriasis tend to have less than optimal vitamin D3, especially in temperate countries.

**Milk Thistle** – Taking 250 milligrams three times daily can reduce cellular growth, as well as help with liver detoxification.

**Zinc** –Zinc is very helpful for the immune system, and in times of sickness the body will try to horde zinc. Since the immune system is always in overdrive with psoriasis, it makes sense to support the immune system and healing. Zinc has been found to be very beneficial in times of sickness and it seems to improve skin outbreaks.

**Vit C**- Vitamin C is a powerful antioxidant and helps with fighting oxidative stress and boosting the immune system, which are both beneficial for Psoriasis.

**Glutamine** – This is an amino acid which has been found to be beneficial to helping with gut repair. Leaky gut and developing a permeable intestinal lining seems to contribute to Psoriasis glutamine can help with healing leaky gut.

# CHAPTER 10

## *Introducing Dietary Changes*

For over 20 years, I suspected that my diet was affecting my skin. I could see that when I ate junk food, flour, sugar, dairy or beef, my skin was redder than normal. Then the opposite would happen when I ate lots of healthy fruits and vegetables. My first indication of the link between diet and Psoriasis came through weight loss.

### Overweight at 220lbs, 37% bodyfat

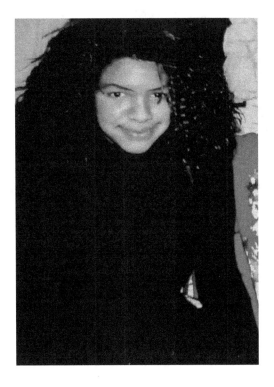

I was over 100Lbs overweight and I was desperate to lose weight and I learned that detoxing my body helped with fat loss. So, I put myself on my first detox program of eating mostly fruits and vegetables, smoothies and lots and lots of water. The first time, it took a long time but, I was shocked because my Psoriasis cleared up 75%. No redness, no itching, very little flaking.

## Losing Over 70 lbs, Weight 150lbs

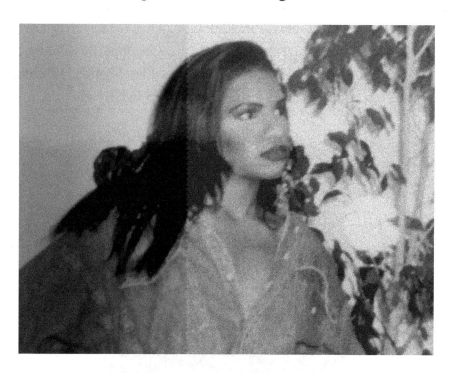

That was my first clue that dietary changes could help to clear my skin. But, as I was new to the process of healthy eating, diet and weight loss, I returned to my old eating habits of consuming alcohol and junk food and psoriasis flared up and spread.

But what I proved, even for a short time was that there was definitely a connection between change in diet and clearing of the skin. I knew that there was a connection. During this period of experimentation, I continued to ask my dermatologist about the possibility that dietary changes could help psoriasis. But, each time, I was told there was no connection between diet and psoriasis. So, I continued to use medications for years, later only to have my skin continue to be flared up over and over.

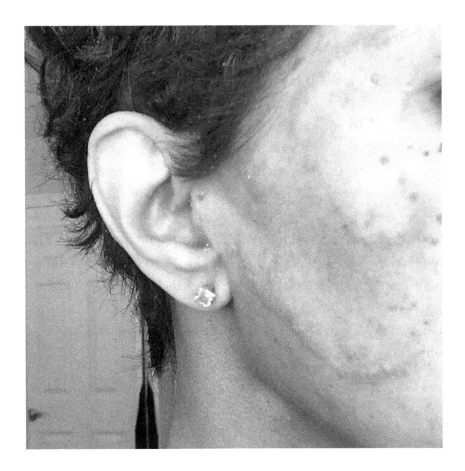

All this time, though my doctors were against it, I was still convinced dietary changes and natural healing could work long term. I had seen it first hand, when my skin cleared with my first detox, so I set out to do my own investigation. I discovered many functional and alternative doctors and naturopaths who support natural healing, and I read all of their works. Dr Pagano was one of the first practitioners to write a book about healing psoriasis with changed diet and lifestyle. Dr. Zoltan Rona, with whom Dr. Pagano collaborated, was in my home city of Toronto, Canada. So now, I knew I was onto something. Dietary changes may not cure psoriasis, but it supports the healing process which happens inside, which leads to a healing of the skin. Dietary changes are suggested for many major conditions like heart disease, diabetes and cancer. So why not psoriasis? I found that many people, in their attempt to heal psoriasis treated it as an allergic reaction, by cutting out one thing or another. Then, weeks later when nothing happened or worse yet the skin got worse with medications; the prevailing belief was that dietary changes did not affect psoriasis. But psoriasis is not an allergy. It's not the body reacting to histamines, which cause psoriasis outbreaks. Psoriasis is an issue with inflammation, the immune system and the liver. So, what we eat can either increase inflammation, or it can decrease inflammation, which in turn affects the immune system and triggers or prevents the healing of psoriasis.

Let's think about why we eat. The human body requires food for nutrients. Food helps the body to function, repairs damage and supports organs, tissues and cells. The amount of nutrition our bodies receives is directly related to how well the digestive system works to extract the needed nutrients. As we have seen, people with psoriasis are likely to have leaky gut which means our digestive system is already underperforming. We also saw that the liver is often under stress, so processing food and nutrition depends on both the digestive system and liver. Next is what are we feeding our bodies. Diet matters. Providing processed food with no nutrients only increases inflammation, making psoriasis worse. Consuming fresh foods, which are anti-inflammatory and fight inflammation, provides the necessary nutrition to help the body heal.

My first step was to take a good look at the foods I was eating and divide them into two categories: inflammatory and anti-inflammatory. The concept behind the Psoriasis Detox Diet is that since the source of psoriasis seems to be in the digestive system, it could be beneficial to psoriasis to consume fresh, anti-inflammatory foods. Since psoriasis is related to inflammation, removing foods that cause inflammation has been shown to support the skin's healing process. Which foods create inflammation? All processed foods, conventional meats, pork, red meat, flour, sugar, dairy and alcohol are inflammatory. Nightshade vegetables have also been found to affect people with psoriasis, so it's important to avoid tomatoes, potatoes, and eggplant.

Psoriasis has been linked to acid alkali balance.

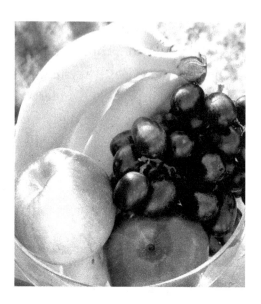

It's very important to increase natural, whole foods like fruits and vegetables. These foods can provide vitamins, minerals and enzymes which help the healing process. I found that making these 70% of my diet, resulted in a major change in the healing time and the appearance of my Psoriasis breakouts.

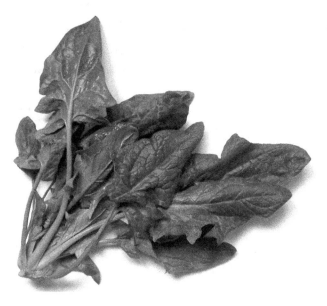

Psoriasis has also been linked to imbalances in bacteria, so it makes sense to consume foods with nutrients like probiotics. Kefir, yogurt, and cultured vegetables can provide good bacteria and help balance bacteria. This practice improves health and improves the appearance of the skin. Psoriasis is also related to oxidation, so increasing antioxidants and alkaline foods has been shown to be very beneficial. Glutathione is the master antioxidant in the body. Increasing this master antioxidant helps to reduce oxidation and free radical damage in the body, so increasing glutathione-building foods is important for people with psoriasis. It is interesting that psoriasis is linked to three major systems in the body, all of which are central to the top diseases – cardiovascular, immune, nervous and detoxification. Reducing oxidation has been shown to improve many of these systems. Onions, asparagus, garlic, cucumbers and more help to build glutathione.

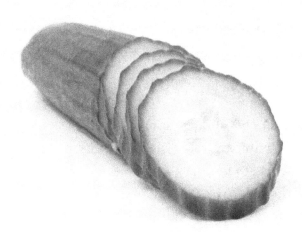

I also increased foods high in anti-oxidants, high in vitamin A like oranges, yellow and dark leafy green vegetables. By adding these winners to your diet on a daily basis, you will increase your **vitamin A**, which is critical for skin healing. Good sources of vitamin A include cantaloupe, carrots, mango, tomatoes, kale, collard greens and watermelon. Antioxidants control oxidation and reduce oxidative damage to tissues and cells.

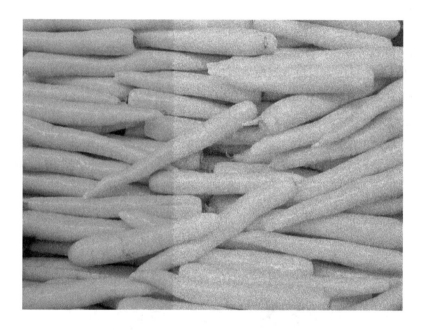

The immune system is central to psoriasis, so I include foods with zinc which is known to boost the immune system. Grass-fed meats, lamb, chickpeas, and pumpkin seeds are also other great sources of zinc. Omega-3 is necessary for every cell in the body and people with psoriasis have been shown to be deficient in Omega-3. Including foods with this nutrient is a great way to improve the condition. Wild-caught fish like salmon, mackerel and sardines are great sources of vitamin D. These should be balanced with foods with Omega 6. Avocados are a great source of Omega 6 and this is a very important nutrient.

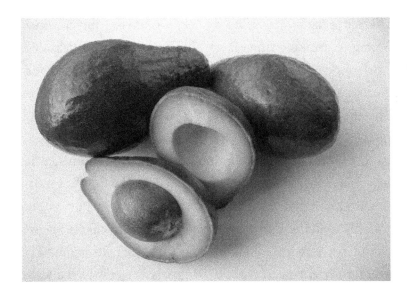

One of the worst things to do during dietary changes is to panic and give up. Introducing toxic food and drink during a detox can trigger a healing crisis causing psoriasis to spread over the body very quickly. I have seen people who are going through steroid withdrawal become frantic when the skin is covered with outbreaks and the healing slows. It's very important to stick to the program and don't give up until you are clear. Once you are completely clear, then you can eat normally. Panic and using medications or creams are not a magic cure and will not work. It simply delays the inevitable—having to use the detox program again and getting the toxins out. Medications are always one choice that you can discuss with your doctor, but in my experience, it is not a long-term solution that leads to completely clear skin, which stays clear.

Dietary changes involves hydration, cutting alcohol and smoking, increasing vegetables and fruit, removing inflammatory foods, getting to sleep by 10 pm, light exercise and stress reduction. There is no cure for psoriasis and even though diet is not a treatment, changes in diet alone can help to support the healing of the body.

The first step to the Psoriasis Detox Diet program is to increase hydration. I recommend drinking three liters of water, which will help in healing from the inside out. After this induction period, the next step is to cut excess carbs, sugar, and dairy while replacing the diet with fruits and veggies. This should be done gradually by substituting a single entity with the healthy diet. The aim is to end up with a diet free from processed food and eat that which has maximum nutrition and minimum calories. This will help relieve the skin and heal properly. Healthy food is fundamental for good health in general. A diet with fewer inflammatory compounds will not only treat but also prevent psoriasis. It may take a few weeks to see the difference, but the long-term accrued benefits should keep you focused on the right diet. I created the Psoriasis Detox Diet after years of experimentation of cutting out foods for periods and incorporating the findings of many natural healers, naturopaths and world-renowned researchers who have uncovered the best practices to support the body's ability to heal. It is extremely important to follow the program until your body heals fully. Natural healing is not like medications or using pharmaceuticals. It involves healing from the inside out, so it takes time.

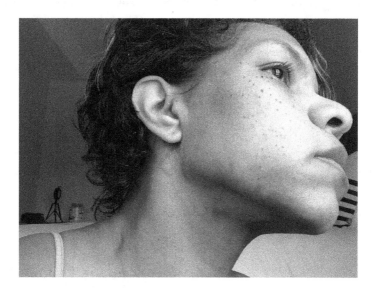

Over the years I have experimented with many diets and while some were specific and helped to heal the skin to 70%, many did not work to completely clear my skin. Many of the re-introduction diets allow re-introduction too early. One of the most important things to do to heal psoriasis is to remove the food and drink, which is inflammatory. Inflammation is one of the major factors which make psoriasis worse. So, until the foods are removed and the inflammation calms down, psoriasis remains impossible to heal. The Psoriasis Detox Diet may seem strict, but it is only through discipline that the body will achieve balance. Cutting this and that food out in a haphazard way only increases stress. When the body is out of harmony, it does not heal. The second thing to understand is that taking pills of any kind, in my experience, did not clear psoriasis without following the diet.

So, supplements alone will not affect the skin as much; however, combined with the right diet and lifestyle factors, they can speed healing. Only when you apply all aspects of the Psoriasis Detox Diet every day will there be significant changes. Healing time varies. Some people who require less cleansing will heal in four weeks; others can take as long as twelve months or longer. Healing time always depends on how much toxins and processed food are consumed. What goes in must come out. If you smoke, consume alcohol, and use medications and steroid creams, expect to take eight to twelve months to heal. If, however, you do not take medications and you follow a relatively clean diet, I have experienced clearing in four to five weeks. In some cases there are added factors and complications like additional medical conditions which can delay healing. Giving your body time to heal is imperative. Nothing worth doing is done in a rush. Healing is long-term and should be treated as an investment in your body's health and future.

# Clear 100% Using Psoriasis Detox Diet

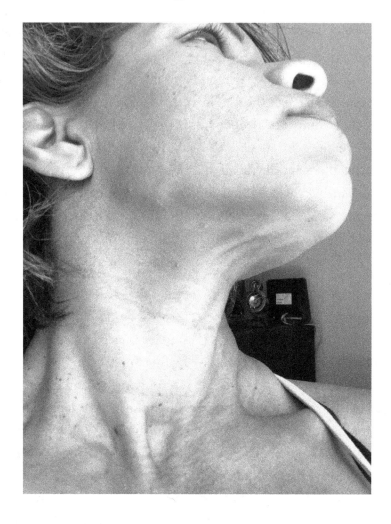

# CHAPTER 11

# The Role of Lifestyle Change

Our lifestyles determine what goes into the body, and that is what gets excreted. Poor lifestyle habits not only lead to psoriatic flare-ups, but they can cause psoriatic arthritis. While psoriasis has no cure, lifestyle modifications can help a great deal in reducing the symptoms and hence improve life in people living with the disease. Lifestyle habits are totally in our control and we decide what to do or eat. Sometimes, it's all about the poor choice of food or drinks when one is faced with the dilemma that variety brings. The changes need not make one strain and live under pressure, but rather there should be small subtractions, adjustments, or additions done over time. As the body allows, you can make more drastic changes and get a better quality of life.

## Manage Stress

Many sources of stress assault the body of an individual suffering from psoriasis. Avoiding the stress agents is advisable, although sometimes it is impossible to do so. If you can't avoid the stressing factors, know how to deal with them. This is the only way to ensure that you remain functional without risking a flare-up of the disease. Identify all the risky things that can worsen your disease and then make a strategic approach to each of them. You can do it on your own or request the help of a friend or a professional. For instance, if cold weather makes your skin dry, it is a potential stressor that will cause a flare-up. You should, therefore, make every effort to ensure that your skin is extra moist during the cold season as you wait for the hot times of the year.

Stress and psoriasis form a vicious cycle in which one makes the other worse. Many people with psoriasis believe that their flare-ups are a result of some form of stress. When they get the symptoms, stress levels increase and the cycle continues. Lowering stress will consequently lower the symptoms of psoriasis. If you can manage your stress well, you can be sure to have a remission of the disease and live without symptoms for a very long time. Knowing what to avoid helps prevent stress and manage it in the future.

## Exercise

Psoriasis can be managed by workouts and meditation exercises. If you are not used to going to the gym, you can start short, with brisk walks and do more with time. Exercise relieves stress that leads to psoriasis. A person who has adopted a form of exercise is more likely to have less stress and lifted spirits together with optimum brain function. Cognitive function is improved with exercise and this determines health. Meditation is scientifically proven to be of benefit in managing stress. People who do yoga or Tai Chi have few cytokines that lead to inflammation.

Psoriatic arthritis and psoriasis gets better when the joints are moved during exercises. Immobility leads to stiffening of the joints in people with this form of arthritis. Water therapy can help one to move effortlessly and for a longer time since the water has no impact on joint movement. This means that you don't have to move as vigorously as you would at the gym. Depending on the part of the body that has pain and joint involvement, you may need to avoid some types of exercise and choose those that are accommodative. Yoga may be the best form of exercise for some people while others can do fine with intense workouts.

## Treat Underlying Diseases

Co-morbidities can make life more difficult for psoriasis sufferers, and the other diseases should be actively treated. Concentrating all your efforts on psoriasis simply because it is more serious won't help much. Making sure that you address obesity, metabolic syndrome, coronary artery disease, and depression, which are common in psoriasis, will help relieve symptoms. Depression can lead to stress, and it has a negative impact on psoriasis management because it affects health-seeking behavior. It will affect motivation for working out and following a healthy lifestyle. Failure to treat all the underlying disease processes makes psoriasis treatment more complicated.

## Eating Healthful Foods

When in pain, one can be quick to look for a food or a drink with lots of sugar because of its rewarding taste. However, this is harmful to people with psoriasis since it will lead to accumulation of excess sugar and cause inflammation. You must stick to a healthy diet that is friendly to psoriasis. Such diets need to be full of anti-oxidants, anti-inflammatory compounds, and nutrients. Alcohol should be taken in moderation or avoided. Alcohol may not affect psoriasis, but it will definitely affect health-seeking behavior and has been shown to interact with psoriasis treatment.

## Stop Smoking

Smoking can be a risk factor for almost any disease. Quitting this habit is helpful in ensuring that medications and interventions for psoriasis work. People who smoke will have problems managing symptoms of psoriasis. Smoking can make all the efforts to stay healthy seem wasted and it is a source of stress to the body's systems.

## Maintain Healthy Weight

You need to maintain a healthy weight if you have psoriasis. Being overweight causes your body to transfer the excess weight to the joints of the lower extremities making psoriatic arthritis worse. Some people lose weight appropriately but regain it because they don't adhere to healthy eating and exercise. Loss of weight is a health intervention that will help your lead a better life with psoriasis. You won't need high doses of drugs for psoriasis if you maintain a healthy weight.

## Get Happy

There is no question that out mental state affects our physical health and well-being. For over twenty years I was depressed, angry and withdrawn, and I believe that this mental state, not only affected my body long-term, but it set up a cycle of stress which continued to contribute to psoriasis outbreaks never healing. Mind body research is done by Candace Pert, who describes how emotions are a series of chemical and chemical reactions affecting the body's systems. This means that people with psoriasis are even more susceptible to physical effects because of the mental stress that dealing with this disease causes daily. As difficult as it is, I found it is important to start each day with an attitude of gratitude. My skin began to change dramatically when I looked at psoriasis as a gift and a wake-up call. Not many people are fortunate enough to have the body warn of impending illness because it is overloaded and unable to handle the stress being placed on it. As soon as I viewed psoriasis as an outward sign of the body pleading for help and as an opportunity to change what I was consuming and my lifestyle, my skin began to heal. I took a positive proactive approach to healing rather than holding negativity and feeling defeated.

# CHAPTER 12

❧

# *The Psoriasis Detox Diet*

fter years of trial and error, my own education, meeting dozens of natural healers and functional doctors and helping thousands of people to clear the skin, I finally created my Psoriasis Detox Diet program. There is no cure for psoriasis, but I found that supporting the healing process, removing toxins and inflammatory foods, cleansing the body and adding nutrients from whole foods helped to clear my skin. Today I am 100% clear and staying clear, almost 4 years later. What's even more wonderful is that thousands of people are following this program today and are achieving incredible results, which they were never able to see previously.

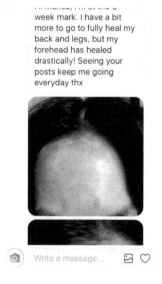

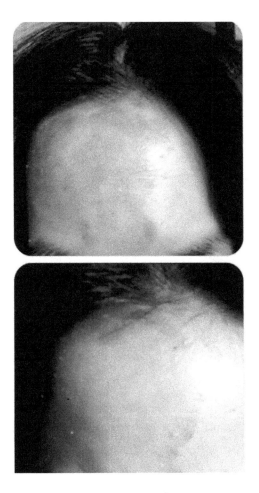

I knew I would always have psoriasis, but because I had it since child-hood, all I wanted was to have clear beautiful skin□no outbreaks and flare-ups. Each person is different. We have different genes, medical histories, backgrounds and all of this can affect healing ability and time. While following the Psoriasis Detox Diet program, I found it was important to take the time to record what works and what doesn't work. I painstakingly listed everything I consumed and put on my skin for years. I tracked every flare-up, clearing time and any other reactions. After doing this long enough, I created the full-program which details all of the steps which must be done daily to result in the improved appearance of the skin.

## Step One – Remove All Toxic Food and Add Water

The first part of my Psoriasis Detox Diet program is to remove all the debris, toxins and bad bacteria which has accumulated and built up in our tissues. Have you ever tried to wash mud off your car after it has built up and caked on. One spray generally is not enough. It requires a diligent effort to scrub off the mud before it's clean. The same is true of the digestive system. Food, toxins and chemicals from junk food build up and they get caked on. The only way to "scrub" the digestive system is to first limit the toxins by cutting out all foods which could affect the body. By reducing the toxins consumed, what is stuck in the digestive system can finally be cleaned out, and we can stop the cycle of consuming processed foods and toxins, which can in turn affect the liver and eventually the skin. Drinking 3 liters of water a day was an important part of this diet. Not only does water help to flush the body of toxins but it helps with hydration and circulation of nutrients throughout the body. I suggest drinking 15 glasses of water a day and maintaining this for one week before moving on to all other steps. Water is so important, even after being clear for years, I continue to drink this much.

## Step Two – Add Lots of Raw Fruits and Vegetables

After this, I added lots of raw vegetables which act as a broom for the intestines. Raw vegetables become an important part of natural heal-ing because of something called insoluble fiber. Fruits and vegetables in general have two types of fiber, soluble and insoluble, but only raw

vegetables have insoluble fiber, which helps to promote proper digestion and elimination and help to sweep the digestive system. This is
the first part of the natural cleansing system.

The Psoriasis Detox Diet program helps to jumpstart the body to
start healing. Raw vegetables also provide good nutrients, which
aid in the healing process. What I found from my own experience
and that of thousands of people with psoriasis is, we tend to eat a
poor diet made up of a lot of cooked, processed food for so many
years that it begins to seriously overwhelm the body's organs and
our health. The body is simply incapable of handling all of the junk,
because with psoriasis, as was shown previously, we are susceptible
to fatty liver disease which means the liver is already compromised
and it is easier to overload it.

The simple act of cutting "trigger foods" for a few days is not enough.
It's also the reason short term detoxes and kits don't work for psoriasis and can make outbreaks worst long-term. First, psoriasis is
not an allergy. Following a strict diet as part of my program helped
to reduce the toxic overload and fuel the body to have the nutrients
needed to heal. But, it is necessary to follow it for a minimum of
sixteen weeks. Only then, will real lasting changes occur. I found
that healing requires a concentrated effort for many weeks sometimes months, to undo all of the damage done for years. The skin
requires proper nutrients and since psoriasis involves many systems,
it is important to consume optimal nutrition to heal them. Even the
slightest bit of overload from medications, toxins, creams, pollution,
bacteria, processed food, gluten and dairy, can prevent the healing
of psoriasis. One of the ways to speed up the healing is by improving elimination. Regular bowel functions are extremely important

for psoriasis as they help to remove the buildup of toxins. Increasing water and fiber contributes tremendously to improving psoriasis and psoriatic arthritis. As part of the Psoriasis Detox Diet program, teas, water, lots of fruits and veggies are all recommended to assist the cleansing process.

## Step 3 – Add Green Smoothies

Liquid nutrition in the form of green smoothies provide nutrients from fruits and vegetables and are an easy way to alleviate stress on the digestive system. Green smoothies made from fruits like banana, blueberries and apples and vegetables like celery, spinach and kale are packed with vitamins, minerals and nutrients. Before starting the Psoriasis Detox Diet, it is best to prepare yourself. You will need to commit to several weeks of restricted eating during the program to see major improvements in the skin and pain reduction.

## Step 4 – Improve Stress Management

Stress management is an extremely important part of the program. As we have seen, psoriasis is linked to stress, so recovery of the body becomes crucial and controlling stress is key. As part of my Psoriasis Detox Diet program, I found it add in activities like meditation, walks in nature and light exercise for stress management.

## Step 5 – Improve Sleep

Sleep is essential for health and even more crucial for people with Psoriasis. Lack of sleep has been shown to have a detrimental effect on the body so getting 7 to 8 hours of deep, uninterrupted sleep is an important part of this program. I found it was best to go to bed by 10PM and wake by 6AM. When my sleep was regulated I saw a tremendous difference in my skin very fast.

## Step 6 – Record Everything and Take Pictures

I found that the best way to begin natural healing is to keeping a journal of everything and take pictures daily. Record everything you consume--the quantities—as well as what activities you did, how you feel and what times you went to bed and woke up. It also helps to track your healing by taking pictures of your skin. Pictures help you to do two things- track your healing and note if for some reason the skin gets worst, it would be possible to refer to what could have been a trigger. I found there were times when I was following the Psoriasis Detox Diet strict and my skin was getting worst. Then I realized by looking at my journal that I was more stressed or I did not have proper sleep or some other factor I had overlooked. Recording everything will help you in the long run. Years later, should Psoriasis be triggered again, you have something to follow and refer to.

Healing Psoriasis is a constant, continuous challenge of figuring out what works for your body. While some people heal extremely fast, others take much longer because we are all individual. It is important to have patience and to stick to healthy habits, no matter the results. I also encourage you to maintain an open conversation with your doctor so, he or she can witness your healing and make extra recommendations. I am 100% healed and never been happier since, following my Psoriasis Detox Diet program.

## 100% Clear and Staying Clear of Psoriasis

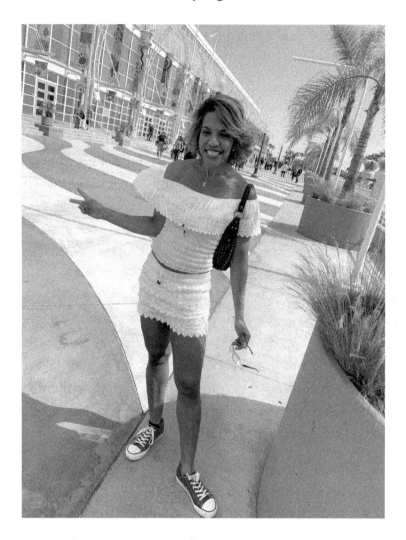

## Re-Introduction of Foods After Completely Clear

Once the skin cleared up completely, this is going to be a period of major happiness. You are going to want to go out more, enjoy life more and stop following the diet. I found that once I was completely I was able to go back to enjoying my favorite foods. But, re-introduction of foods must be done super slowly.

## Week 1 - Completely Clear

Continue to drink 15 glasses of water and drink one green smoothie and eat one big salad but for dinner you may introduce foods like – quinoa tomatoes, potatoes and peppers. Whole foods which were previously on the DO NOT eat list. Do this by adding one in for dinner.

## Week 2 – Completely Clear (Add Nightshades)

Continue to Add in Foods and drink 15 glasses of water as well as drink one green smoothie and eat one big salad. Now you can add in nightshades as well as nuts and seeds.

**Week 3 and Week 4** -Keep up this diet without adding anything else in.

**Week 5** – Completely Clear (Add Beef and Flour)

If you are still completely clear you may add in beef, eggs, noodles and one meal with flour in it. For example – pasta or bread. Along with the nightshades, nuts and seeds and still having a green smoothie and one big salad a day.

**Week 6 and Week 7** – Continue following the same diet.

**Week 8** – Eat Normal

If you are still completely clear my suggestion is to keep up a green smoothie in the morning and one big salad a day but you can now eat normal foods which were previously on the DO NOT EAT list. You may also add in one or two alcoholic drinks ONCE a week.

The Psoriasis Detox Diet helped me to clear my skin and today, almost 4 years later, I am remaining clear. However, I know that, because there is no cure for Psoriasis, at any moment it is possible that psoriasis can be triggered again. The important benefit of having cleared the skin once is you now have a roadmap to use forever along with your detailed notes and record. If I ever have another flare-up I will know exactly what to do. So, far so good. It's been over three years and I am clear and staying clear. No sign of outbreaks.

There are six steps to this program and all must be done daily for the best results

1. Maintain Hydration.

2. Maintain Alkaline/Acid balance.

3. Consume whole foods.

4. Take supplements.

5. Exercise positivity and stress management.

6. Get adequate sleep.

I found that if I addressed all six steps each day, I had optimal results and my psoriasis healed quicker. The key to this program is to stick to it as strictly as you can. This can be a challenge because we are essentially forming new habits for diet and lifestyle. Breaking old habits can be a challenge, but it is worth it in the end to see the skin healing and outbreaks fading.

Food is a crucial part of the Psoriasis Detox Diet and it helped me to identify my habits with food and consuming a lot of junk. It forced me to take stock and to realize that ¾ of what I was consuming was toxic processed food which only made my skin worst. Since these habits were ingrained since childhood, to change my eating felt impossible. But, I knew in order to take control of psoriasis, I had to take control of my food intake. I believe this is the most crucial part. Food heals and food kills. There is no dispute about food which contributes to the onset of diabetes and heart disease, so it was not surprising that I could see the effects on psoriasis.

Inflammatory foods contribute to all disease, so once they are cut, there will be an improvement in the skin within three to four weeks, with full clearing possible by eight to twelve weeks. What you need to know, though, is that natural healing works with your body's needs and ability to heal, and the speed of healing is individual. We all have complex genes and medical and family histories, so this--together with the amount of toxins consumed, the amount of medications used, type of psoriasis and lifestyle--all play a part in the healing process. It is necessary to work with your body and give it the time it needs to heal. I cleared in six weeks, but this was after fifteen years of trial and error and numerous detoxes and cleanses. Others take three to four months; still others heal in six to eight months. Healing time varies, but supporting the healing process with dietary changes and natural remedies always has positive effects for 99% of people with psoriasis. In fact the 1% who didn't see results, generally admitted they had no willpower to follow the program. And, it's okay, because when you are ready to heal, I found that it becomes a much simpler process with less resistance.

By removing inflammatory foods, remove the triggers and give the skin a chance to heal.

**The most inflammatory foods and drink are as follows**

- Alcohol

- Smoking

- Soda and smoking

- Packaged foods

- Flour

- Dairy

- Gluten

- Sugar

- Nightshades –tomatoes, potatoes

# Foods To Cut Out- Do Not Eat List

The following foods seem to affect psoriasis:

## 1. Alcohol

Alcohol is one of the worst things for psoriasis, and I found that not only was I required to eliminate alcohol, but I had to *wait four weeks* before my skin began to heal. Alcohol affects the liver and it causes inflammation, so it's not surprising that it is among the top substances which affect psoriasis.

## 2. Gluten

Gluten has been found to cause many digestive disorders, so it's no surprise that it affects psoriasis. The issue with gluten is that it is hidden in many foods including bread, pasta, pizza, cakes, pies, sandwiches, wraps, cereals, chips, crackers and more. I found it best to cut out all packaged foods so I didn't accidentally consume any of it. Gluten is extremely inflammatory and psoriasis may take a couple of days to flare up after eating it, but eating even small amounts of gluten prevents the complete healing of my skin.

### 3. Nuts and Seeds

Nuts and seeds are normally very healthy. Many vegans consume lots of nuts and seeds, but I found that eating nuts and seeds triggered psoriasis and made it impossible to heal completely. The gut is inflamed when the skin flares up, so I think that nuts and seeds are hard on the digestive system, which is why I believe it affects psoriasis.

### 4. Citrus

Citrus fruits--oranges limes tangerines and grapefruit--have been shown to affect some people, so I found it necessary to eliminate them. Oranges and tangerines also have a lot of sugar, and since psoriasis is correlated with excess intake of sugar, I found that my skin healed much faster if I eliminated it.

### 5. Soy and Soy Oil

Soy has been found to increase inflammation and affect estrogen. So, since psoriasis is made worse by inflammation, avoid soy and soy oil.

### 6. Milk

Milk is very acidic and many people are lactose intolerant. Since psoriasis is linked to acid alkali balance, I found that it was important to avoid it. Milk and dairy products have been found to contain hormones, which are passed from animals to humans. Since all toxicity will affect psoriasis, it is important to avoid milk until the skin heals.

### 7. Eggs

Eggs have been found to affect some people and eggs tend to make allergic reactions worse. Even though psoriasis is not an allergy, I found it necessary to cut down on anything to which I have a sensitivity. So, I suggest limiting eggs to once a week.

## 8. Fried Foods

Fried foods have been found to be carcinogenic, so it's not surprising that they have been found to affect psoriasis. Fried foods generally have little to no nutrition, so they will never support the healing of the skin and could potentially trigger a flare up. I eliminate all fries, fried chicken, vegetables, seafood, fritters etc. from my diet.

## 9. Nightshades

Nightshade vegetables have been found to affect some people with psoriasis. They contain lectins, which are poisonous compounds used to repel insects. Nightshades like tomato, potato, eggplant and peppers should be eliminated until the skin heals.

## 10. Sugar

Psoriasis has been linked to cardiovascular disease and diabetes, so excessive sugar consumption has been found to cause psoriasis flare-ups. In fact many functional doctors suggest cutting sugar from the diet for a few weeks. I found that it was easier to maintain the diet, but eliminate processed sugar including soda, candy, ice-cream, and all packaged products including sauces and condiments.

# Psoriasis Detox Diet

## Recipes

The following are helpful recipes for foods which are Psoriasis friendly. Please continue to track your results to see what works for your individual body.

## SMOOTHIES

### Baby Spinach, Celery and Banana Smoothie

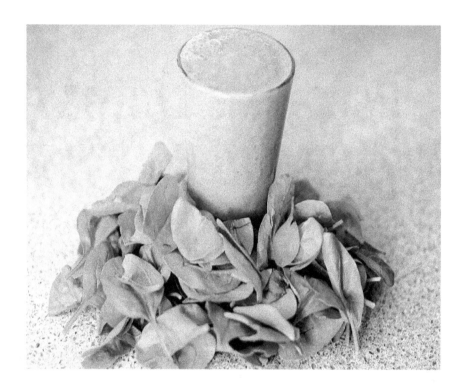

# Baby Spinach, Celery and Banana Smoothie Cont'd

Ingredients:

- 1 cup of baby spinach, cleaned

- ½ cup of water

- 1 banana cut up

- ½ cup of water

Method:

1. In a blender, add all the ingredients.

2. Blend the mixture thoroughly.

3. Serve chilled.

# Fruits and Vegetable Smoothie

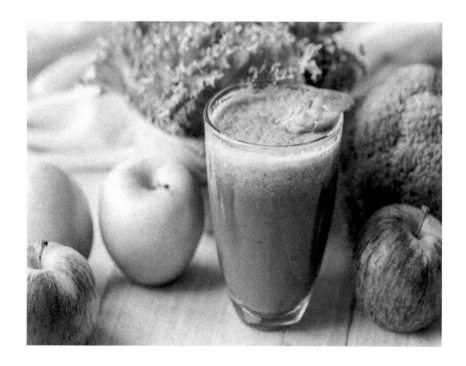

# *Fruits and Vegetable Smoothie Cont'd*

Ingredients:

- 1 green apple, cleaned and cubed
- 1 cup of kale, cleaned
- ¼ cup of broccoli, cleaned
- ½ red apple, cleaned and cubed
- 1 cup of water

Method:

1. In a blender, add all the ingredients.
2. Blend the mixture thoroughly.
3. Serve chilled.

# Kiwi with Mint Smoothie

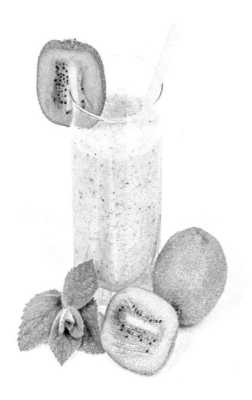

# Kiwi with Mint Smoothie Cont'd

Ingredients:

- 1 cup of kiwi, cleaned and sliced

- 2 tbsp mint leaves, chopped

- 1 banana cut up

- ½ cup of water

Method:

1. In a blender, add all the ingredients.

2. Blend the mixture thoroughly.

3. Serve chilled.

# Apricots and Ginger Smoothie

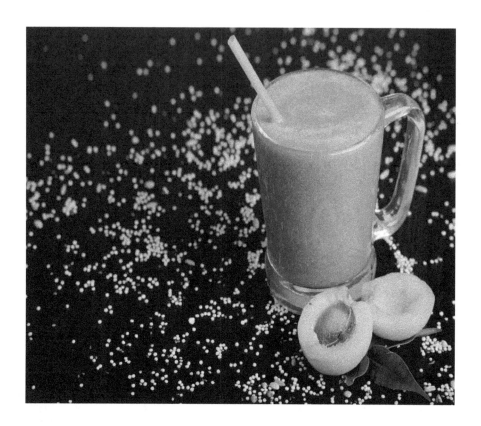

# Apricots and Ginger Smoothie Cont'd

Ingredients:

- ½ cup of apricots

- 1 tbsp of ginger, chopped

- 1 cup of water

- ¼ tbsp of honey

Method:

1. In a blender, add all the ingredients.

2. Blend the mixture thoroughly.

3. Serve chilled.

## BREAKFAST

*Omelette*

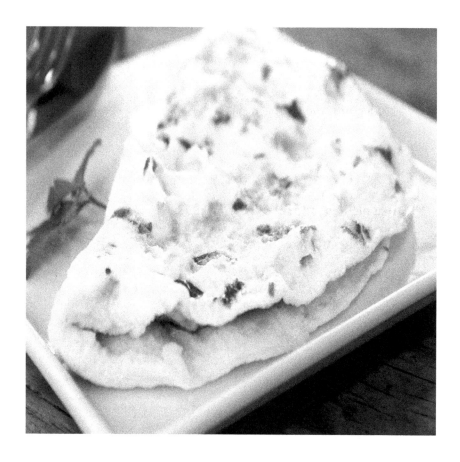

# Omelette Cont'd

Ingredients:

- 3 eggs
- 1 tbsp of parsley, finely chopped
- 1 tbsp of lemon grass, chopped
- ½ tbsp of thyme
- ½ tbsp of turmeric powder
- 1 tbsp of freshly ground pepper
- 1 tbsp of olive oil
- Salt to taste

Method:

1. In a bowl, add all the ingredients except olive oil.
2. Give a thorough mix using an electric beater.
3. In a hot pan, add olive oil and egg mixture.
4. Cook at low heat with lid on. Serve hot.

# Mushroom Omelette

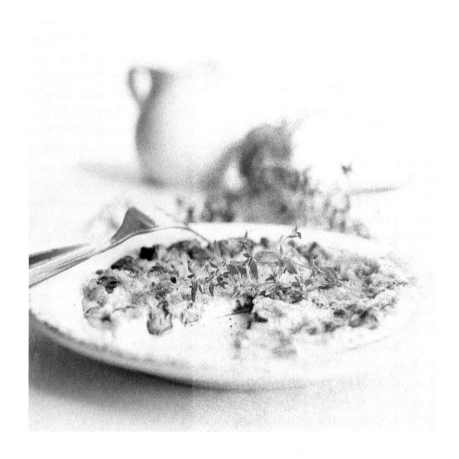

# Mushroom Omelette Cont'd

## Ingredients:

- 3 eggs

- ¼ cup of mushroom, cut into small pieces

- ½ tbsp of thyme

- A pinch of turmeric powder

- 1 tbsp of freshly ground pepper

- 1 tbsp of olive oil

- Salt to taste

## Method:

1. In a bowl, add all the ingredients except olive oil.

2. Mis thoroughly using an electric beater.

3. In a hot pan, add olive oil and egg mixture.

4. Cook at low heat with lid on. Serve hot.

## SALADS

### Boiled Chicken with Green Salad

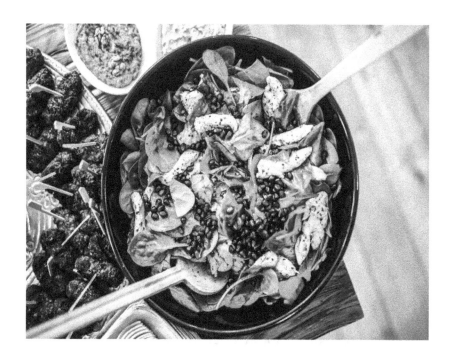

# Chicken with Green Salad

Ingredients:

- 1 cup of spinach leaves, cleaned

- ½ cup of chicken pieces, Pan cooked or baked

- ¼ cup of pomegranate seeds

- 1 tbsp of oregano

- ½ tbsp of lime juice

- 1 tbsp of freshly ground black pepper

- Salt to taste

Method:

1. Cook chicken and cool.

2. Add all the ingredients to a bowl.

3. Mix thoroughly.

4. Serve.

# Greens and Avocado Mix

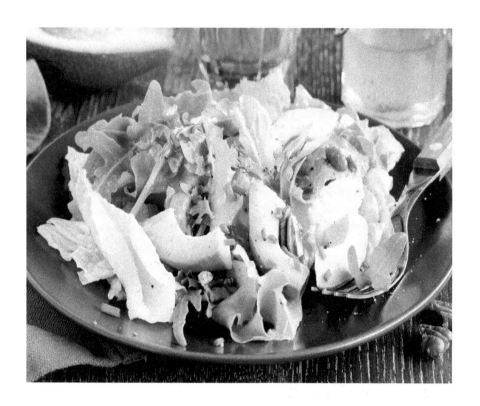

# Greens and Avocado Mix Cont'd

Ingredients:

- 1 cup of arugula leaves
- ¼ cup of green cabbage leaves, cut into small pieces
- ¼ cup of lettuce, cut into small pieces
- ¼ cup of avocado slices
- 1 tbsp of walnuts
- ½ tbsp of freshly ground pepper
- ¼ tbsp of lemon juice
- Salt to taste

Method:

1. In a bowl, add all the ingredients and mix thoroughly.
2. Serve.

# Chicken and Veggie Mix

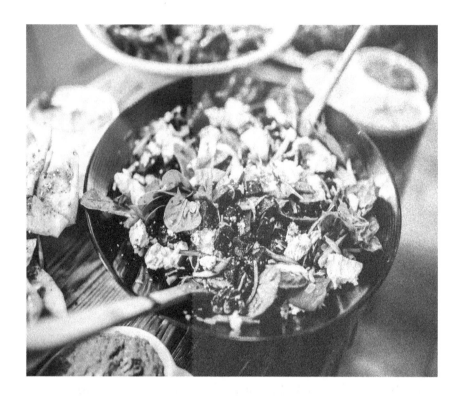

# Chicken and Veggie Mix

**Ingredients:**

- 1 cup of beet root pieces, steamed
- ½ cup of chicken pieces, steamed
- 1 cup of baby spinach leaves, cleaned
- 1 tbsp of freshly ground pepper
- ¼ tbsp of orange juice
- Salt to taste

**Method:**

1. Mix all ingredients in a large bowl.
2. Mix thoroughly and serve.

# Steamed Broccoli with Veggies

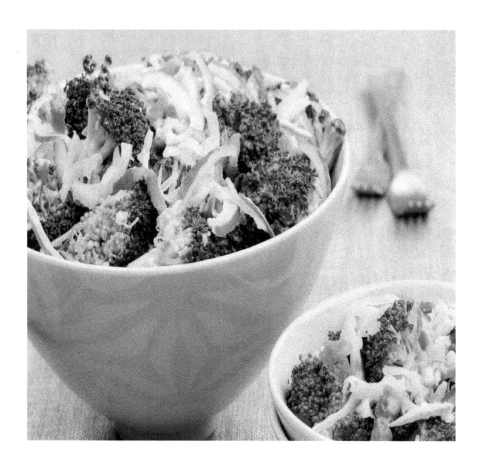

# *Steamed Broccoli with Veggies Cont'd*

Ingredients:

- 1 cup of broccoli florets, steamed
- ¼ cup of spaghetti squash, grated
- ½ onion, sliced
- 1 tbsp of orange juice
- ½ tbsp of freshly ground black pepper
- Salt to taste

Method:

1. Place all ingredients in a bowl.
2. Mix gently mix.
3. Serve fresh.

# Steamed Butternut Squash

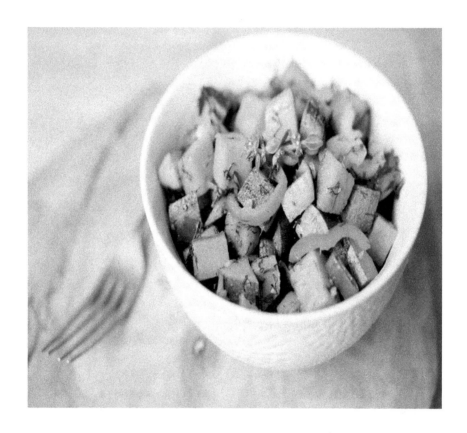

# Steamed Butternut Squash Cont'd

Ingredients:

- 1 cup of butternut squash, cubed and steamed
- 1 slice of pepper cut up (If sensitive leave it out)
- ¼ cup of yam chunks, steamed
- 2 tbsp of spring onions chopped
- 1 tbsp of thyme
- ½ tbsp of oregano
- Salt

Method:

1. Mix all of the ingredients in a bowl thoroughly.
2. Serve fresh.

# Stuffed Grape Leaves and Olives

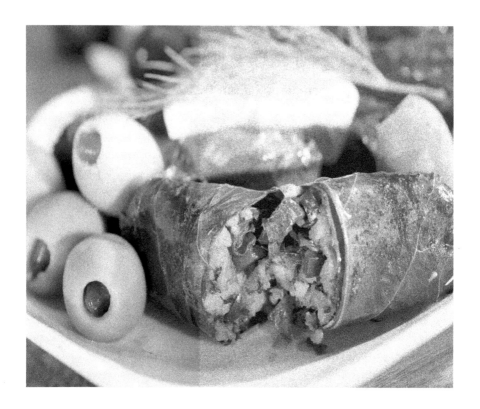

# Stuffed Grape Leaves and Olives

Ingredients:

- 2-3 grape leaves
- 1 cup of seedless green olive
- ¼ cup of salmon pieces
- 1 cup of boiled sweet potatoes
- ½ cup of chopped spinach
- 1 tbsp of ginger-garlic paste
- 1 tbsp of chopped red bell pepper
- 1 tbsp of ground pepper
- Salt

Method:

1. In a bowl, combine salmon pieces and salt.
2. Mix thoroughly.
3. Stuff these olives with salmon pieces.
4. In a bowl, add boiled sweet potatoes and smash with a fork.
5. Add ginger-garlic paste, red bell pepper, spinach, pepper and salt.
6. Mix thoroughly.
7. Spread the grapes leaves and add sweet potato mixture to one end of grape leaf and roll it.
8. Steam stuffed grape leaves for about 20 min.
9. Serve hot with stuffed olives.

# Steamed Broccoli and Mushroom

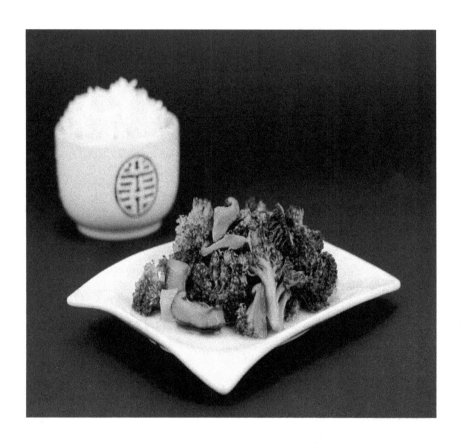

# Steamed Broccoli and Mushroom Cont'd

## Ingredients:

- ½ cup of broccoli florets

- ½ cup of mushroom slices

- 1 tbsp of freshly ground pepper

- 1 tbsp of honey

- Salt to taste

## Method:

1. Combine ingredients in a bowl.

2. Mix thoroughly.

3. Transfer the content to a steamer.

4. Steam the veggies for 10 min.

5. Serve hot.

**SNACKS**

## Spicy Avocado Cream

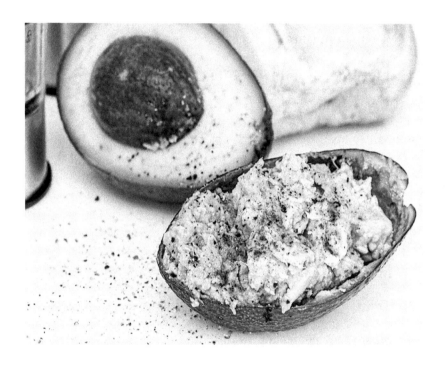

# Spicy Avocado Cream Cont'd

Ingredients:

- 1 avocado

- 1 tbsp of paprika powder

- ¼ tbsp of freshly ground pepper

- ¼ tbsp of cinnamon powder

- Salt to taste

Method:

1. Cut the avocado in two.

2. Remove the seeds and smash the avocado in in the shell.

3. Add paprika powder, ground pepper, cinnamon powder and salt.

4. Give a quick mix.

5. Serve.

# Crispy Anchovies

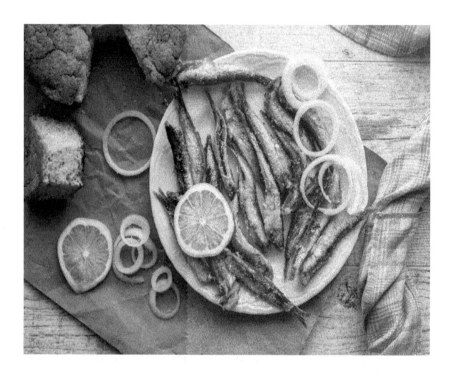

# Crispy Anchovies Cont'd

Ingredients:

- 350 g of anchovies, cleaned
- 1 tbsp of turmeric powder
- ¼ tbsp of garlic powder
- ½ tbsp of lemon juice
- ½ tbsp of olive oil
- Salt to taste

Method:

1. Combine all the ingredients and mix thoroughly.
2. Allow the mixture to sit for 1 hour.
3. After 1 hour, transfer the anchovies to a baking tray.
4. Bake at 180C for 25 min.
5. Serve hot.

# Radish and Potato Hash Browns

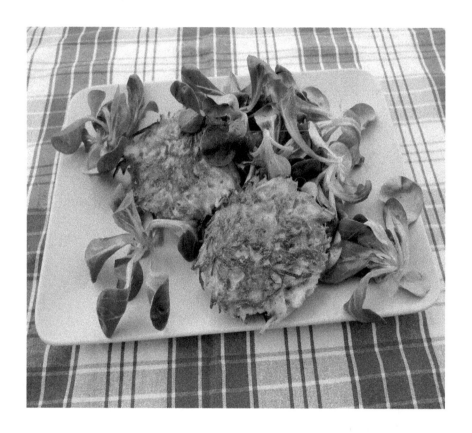

# Radish and Potato Hash Browns Cont'd

**Ingredients:**

- 1 cup of grated radish
- ½ cup of grated potato
- ½ tbsp of ground pepper
- 1 tbsp of grape seed oil
- Salt

**Method:**

1. In a bowl, combine ingredients except grape seed oil.
2. Mix and make into hash browns.
3. Grease the baking tray with grape seed oil.
4. Bake at 200C for 25 min.
5. Serve hot.

# Sweet Potato & Calamari Soup

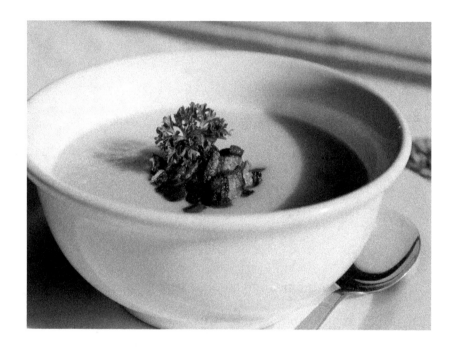

# Sweet Potato & Calamari Soup

Ingredients:

- 1 cup of sweet potato,

- ½ cup of calamari

- 1 tbsp of ground pepper

- 2 tbsp of thyme

- 1 cup of fish stock water

- Salt

Method:

1. Combine ingredients in a soup vessel.

2. Add stock water and cover.

3. Allow the mixture to boil for 10 min.

4. Turn off the heat and allow the mixture to cool down.

5. Blend the mixture until it reaches smooth consistency.

6. Serve.

# Pumpkin and Anchovie Soup

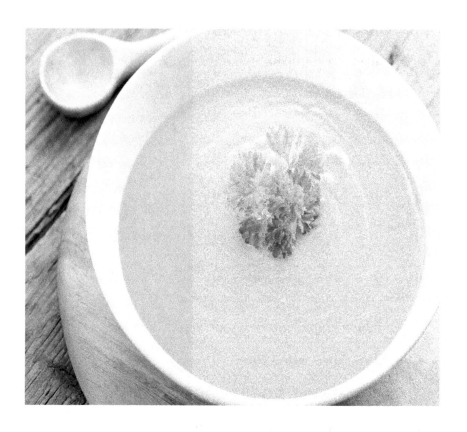

# *Pumpkin and Anchovie Soup Cont'd*

Ingredients:

- 1 cup of pumpkin, cubes
- 200g of anchovies steamed and bones removed
- ½ cup of white onions
- 1 tbsp of olive oil
- 1 tbsp of lime juice
- Salt to taste

Method:

1. In a soup vessel, combine pumpkin, anchovies, white onions and salt.
2. Sauté for 5 min.
3. Add 2 cups of water and put the lid on.
4. Boil for 10-15 min.
5. Turn off the heat and allow the mixture to cool.
6. Blend the pumpkin mixture until it reaches smooth consistency.
7. Serve hot.

# Kale and Spinach Soup

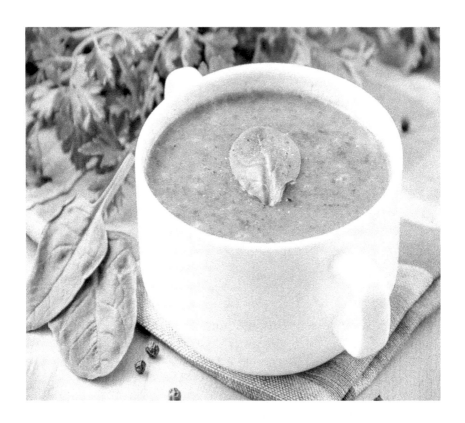

# Kale and Spinach Soup Cont'd

Ingredients:

- 1 cup of baby spinach leaves

- ½ cup of kale leaves

- 1 cup of chicken stock water

- 1 tbsp of ground pepper

- 1 tbsp of lemon juice

- Salt

Method:

1. In a soup vessel, combine ingredients except lemon juice and bring the mixture to boil.

2. Boil for at least 10 min.

3. Turn off the heat and allow the mixture to cool.

4. Add the spinach mixture to a blender and blend them thoroughly.

5. Add lemon juice and serve.

CPSIA information can be obtained
at www.ICGtesting.com
Printed in the USA
LVHW081358101220
673836LV00042B/836